CRYSTALS, FABRICS, AND FIELDS

Crystals, Fabrics, and Fields

*Metaphors of Organicism in
Twentieth-Century Developmental Biology*

Donna Jeanne Haraway

New Haven and London, Yale University Press, 1976

Library of Congress catalog card number: 75-18174
International standard book number: 0-300-01864-9

Designed by Susan McCrillis Kelsey
and set in Baskerville type.
Printed in the United States of America by
The Murray Printing Co., Forge Village, Massachusetts.

Published in Great Britain, Europe, and Africa by
Yale University Press, Ltd., London.
Distributed in Latin America by Kaiman & Polon,
Inc., New York City; in Australasia by Book & Film
Services, Artarmon, N.S.W., Australia; in India by
UBS Publishers' Distributors Pvt., Ltd., Delhi;
in Japan by John Weatherhill, Inc., Tokyo.

To
G. Evelyn Hutchinson
for his inspiration and encouragement at every turn

Contents

Acknowledgments

Many persons have helped in the writing of this book. Their intellectual, emotional, and material support is deeply appreciated. I wish especially to thank G. Evelyn Hutchinson, E. J. Boell, F. L. Holmes, R. S. Brumbaugh, Joseph Needham, Paul Weiss, C. H. Waddington, J. H. Woodger, June G. Goodfield, P. G. Werskey, Carolyn van Heukelem, Richard Stith, and the Danforth Foundation.

Two special friends are responsible for the warmth and space to work. They are Jaye Miller and Helen Woods.

Paradigm and Metaphor

To cast off the rotten rags of memory by inspiration,
To cast off Bacon, Locke, and Newton from Albion's covering,
To take off his filthy garments and clothe him with imagination;
To cast aside from poetry all that is not inspiration,
That it no longer shall dare to mock with the aspersion of madness
Cast on the inspired by the tame high finisher of paltry blots
Indefinite or paltry rhymes, or paltry harmonies, . . .
Who pretend to poetry that they may destroy imagination
By imitation of nature's images drawn from remembrance

William Blake

If the history of science were a disinterested, purely descriptive account of objective operations performed to elucidate the workings of a nature no one believed in anymore, it would raise few passions. Similarly, if science were progressive in the sense of an ever enlarging body of true statements about an ever unchanging yet fundamentally inaccessible world, nature would be seen simply as a big puzzle to be solved. Surely there would be no fundamental insights into personal or historical experience to be expected from pursuing such a science. Simple cumulative science would be a curse. Those with leisure, money, and arbitrary reason to solve puzzles could devote their time to it. They could then present solutions to society, which would translate them into technology in the interests of current power alignments, benign or otherwise. History would be the search into the past for the truly clever who anticipated the later, better solutions to problems. But at the same time, the hope of approaching nearer and nearer to nature is not surrendered lightly in science. Nor should it be. If the views of science espoused both by the old realists and by the more recent positivists are to be rejected, it remains for us to understand in what sense science is progressive and in what way it might lead to an

appreciation of the structure of nature. It seems that the task of contemporary history and philosophy of science is to rediscover for this
age a humane sense of scientific research and theory. For it is a fact
that the history of science does raise passions, and the basic perspective
adopted toward the status of scientific worlds does condition our
poetry and our politics. Surely much of our dis-ease with modern
science comes from appreciation of the inadequacy of the old view of
progressive, control-oriented, objective descriptions of nature (or of
meter readings, if nature herself is hiding or dead).

Two fundamental problems in understanding science can be noted:
How does science change and what are the implications of the view
adopted for the theoretical corpus of a science? Second, in what way
can a science lead to a sense of the natural? To approach these two
very broad issues, it is useful to look at a quite restricted area of one
science, developmental biology, in the first half of the twentieth
century. The period is a time of basic crisis in which the age-old
dichotomy between mechanism and vitalism was reworked and a
fruitful synthetic organicism emerged, with far-reaching implications
for experimental programs and for our understanding of the structure
of organisms. As a key aid in analyzing a period of change in a science,
it is instructive to explore the notion of a paradigm as applied to
biology. The book by Thomas Kuhn, *The Structure of Scientific Revolutions*
(1962), is of central importance in exploring a change in a biological
paradigm. An important aspect of a paradigm is metaphor, and it is
suggestive to investigate the use of metaphor to direct research and its
interpretation. The paradigm concept is rich with suggestions for
analyzing the proper place of metaphor in biology. To begin to understand again the place of image in a science should suggest a way in
which natural structure can be seen in a post-positivist age.[1] Visual
imagery in particular is of critical importance.

---

1. Kuhn himself does not believe that science "draws constantly nearer to some goal set by
nature in advance." The progressive aspect of science is different for him. "Can we not account for
both science's existence and its success in terms of evolution *from* [emphasis added] the community's state of knowledge at any given time? Does it really help to imagine that there is some one
full, objective, true account of nature and that the proper measure of scientific achievement is the
extent to which it brings us closer to that ultimate goal?" (1962, p. 170). The view to be developed
below is different from Kuhn's but it is through his discussion of paradigm and paradigm communities that this study will approach the problem of natural structures. This essay will not be able
to discuss adequately many important issues raised by Kuhn. For a relevant critique see Kordig
1971.

Kuhn raises a host of interesting problems when he introduces the notion of paradigm change. Normal science, he claims, proceeds by exploring the suggestions derived from a dominant paradigm. The paradigm is not a set of explicit rules of procedure but rather "an object for further articulation and specification under new or more stringent conditions" (p. 23). Kuhn simply takes a device common to writers of history, the period, and applies it to a field thought to have developed differently from the rest of human endeavor, that is, in a straight line with occasional Dark Ages and metaphysical sidetracks. But his deeper value lies in refining two aspects of scientific paradigm: paradigm as shared constellation of belief (or disciplinary matrix) and paradigm as model or example. Both the communal and the exemplar nature of paradigms are essential to understanding fundamental change in a science.

The first aspect leads to a consideration of particular communities in science, their formation and modes of communication, and their types of interaction with conflicting scientific communities using different images and thus different languages. Kuhn's book has been criticized as leading to a highly subjective view of science in which an undefinable central picture conditioned all activity and prevented the believer from talking with any but the converted (Lakatos and Musgrave 1970). Thus the paradigm could be shown but not rigorously defined. The distinction is not far from that made by Wittgenstein in his *Tractatus* between saying and showing. Science might become more poetic in the mind of the general public if such a belief were widely held, but would it be any more intelligible? Kuhn argues, however, that his view is more historically accurate for describing what real scientists have done. Further, it is not open to the charge of subjectivity because paradigms and their constituent metaphors are eminently community possessions whose principal value lies in their growing points. In contrast, a view of scientific theory that does not give a large place to metaphor, with its predictive value and potential for development, has trouble accounting for the very progressive aspect of science such views are most often interested in.

If one feels he has a strong support for a view of objective science (i.e. separable from the historical context in which the science developed and separable from any heuristic props used in getting to pure formal theory) he will naturally feel that Kuhn's view of science is dangerously relativistic. In the second edition of *The Structure of Scientific Revolutions*

(1970), Kuhn answers such charges by refining his meaning of *community*. More is shared than the articulated theories. A whole system of assumptions, values, and techniques is involved. Paradigm as disciplinary matrix involves sharing (1) symbolic generalizations that give points of attachment for using logical and mathematical techniques in solving puzzles of normal science; (2) belief in the appropriateness of particular models, such as fields or atoms in a void; (3) values about such things as the place of prediction in an explanation; and (4) exemplars or concrete typical solutions used in the literature and important to the formation of students. Kuhn recognizes degrees of assent, and discerning the fine structure of paradigm groups would involve constructing a thorough sociology of science.

A simpler approach to community will be sufficient for the purposes of this essay. In looking at a time of paradigm change in developmental biology, it is important to note the types of association of biologists involved in the revolutionary switch of metaphor. The Theoretical Biology Club in the 1930s in Cambridge, England, is a suggestive example. Members of the group were interested in bringing to biology the power of logic and mathematical explanation previously enjoyed in the physical sciences, but they were not merely a modern variant of workers operating on a mechanistic paradigm. They shared also the view that hierarchical organization, form, and development were the central concerns of a new biology. Sensing a crisis and sharing a view of the future, the club self-consciously tried to make explicit among themselves the implications of their views. Its members were importantly involved in the transition to an organismic, nonvitalist paradigm for developmental biology.

A second example from biology of an emerging paradigm community of the same period is that of the crystallographers turning attention to biological molecules.[2] Their attitudes and experimental work were significant in the critical refocusing of the relations of physics to biology and of biochemistry to morphology. A present-day paradigm group sharing the organismic paradigm that was born in its current form in the first half of this century is the Alpbach group.

2. John Law of the Science Studies Unit of the University of Edinburgh is doing an extremely provocative study of the paradigm community of British crystallographers of the 1930s and beyond. It would be hard to overestimate the importance of this group for the course of developmental and molecular biology. The enrichment of concepts of structure in molecules was a major ingredient in brewing a nonvitalist organicism.

Participants in the Alpbach Symposium of 1968 include a former member of the Theoretical Biology Club, C. H. Waddington.[3] His relationship to the group, however, was tenuous, largely due to divergent views on mechanisms of heredity. Neither the Alpbach group nor the TBC represent tight working groups from closely related laboratories. Instead, they represent scientists groping toward a common metaphor appropriate across several previously separate areas of science. Their disagreements are as revealing as their agreements. The nature of the community forming upon the transformation of the vitalistic–mechanistic controversy will need more sensitive attention later. It is enough here to note that a shared paradigm is more than an aesthetic predisposition peculiar to a few minds. It is a concrete, common picture of the central focus of a science. The picture conditions the problems seen by the community and the types of solutions admitted as legitimate. The problem for this study is to sketch the picture and to point out subtle but important differences in the paradigm core for various workers.

In addition to stressing the community nature of paradigms, Kuhn's thesis is fruitful in another sense. The process of switch of paradigm is compared to a revolution. A major reorientation of fundamental metaphor occurs, leading workers in a field to see new problems and to accept radically different sorts of explanations. Normal science is characterized by the solution of puzzles, a truly cumulative enterprise, made possible by "a strong network of commitments—conceptual, theoretical, instrumental, and methodological" (Kuhn 1970, p. 42). By contrast,

> the transition from a paradigm in crisis to a new one from which a new tradition of normal science can emerge is far from a cumulative process, one achieved by an articulation or extension of the old paradigm. Rather it is a reconstruction of the field from new fundamentals, a reconstruction that changes some of the field's most elementary theoretical generalizations as well as many of its paradigm methods and applications. [Kuhn 1970, p. 84]

3. See Koestler and Smythies 1969; the book is based on papers and discussion of the Alpbach symposium. Among the participants were Ludwig von Bertalanffy, Jean Piaget, Barbel Inhelder, Paul Weiss, and W. H. Thorpe. Weiss and Waddington have long been divided on important biological issues, and these divisions were also apparent at the meetings.

If such is the case, normal science must be particularly good at generating periods of crisis in which the switches will occur. Kuhn points out that the perception of anomaly is the first step in the production of full-scale crisis. The paradigm inspires certain expectations. If such expectations repeatedly are not met, strains are introduced into the total paradigm system. Kuhn's historical examples of anomaly and crisis in science are drawn from chemistry and physics. The phlogiston theory led workers to expect metals to behave in a particular way when roasted. Experiments with the red oxide of mercury did not fulfill such anticipations. Perception of the anomaly alone was not sufficient to lead to the discovery of oxygen, but it was critical that the problems presented by the old paradigm were proving resistant to proper solution. The paradigm was failing in application to its own traditional problems (Kuhn 1970, p. 69).

There is an illuminating biological parallel to the examples given by Kuhn. The strict atomistic, mechanistic paradigm applied to organisms led Driesch in 1891 to expect the echinoderm egg to behave like a good machine. That is, its development should have been "mosaic": the parts should have their fates fixed at the outset and simple interaction of atomic parts according to mechanical laws should be the essence of development. Regulation was not an admissible occurrence within a strict mechanistic paradigm. Driesch formed his expectations in such allegiance to the paradigm that he was certain his experiment of killing one of the first two blastomeres resulting from the first cleavage of sea urchin eggs would result in half-embryos. The appearance of whole little animals in his dish precipitated a practical and philosophic crisis of the first rank in embryology. The old paradigm seals its own fate by the operation of its own dynamic.

Two further aspects of paradigm change can be drawn from the example of Driesch. Kuhn notes that periods of crisis and revolution are marked by concern over the philosophic foundations of the science not evident in times of normal functioning. Ordinary scientists, used to a certain degree of confidence in their epistemological and metaphysical commitments, come to feel a need to defend their positions or to evolve new ones. The first third of this century was marked by constant debates between neomechanists, neovitalists, and older brands of each. Despite the fact that each camp rested secure in the belief that reason and experiment resided with it alone, no resolution could or did occur until the machine paradigm common to mechanist and vitalist alike was fundamentally altered; the metaphor was of central relevance. Thus the second aspect of Kuhn's analysis of paradigm change:

> The act of judgment that leads scientists to reject a previously accepted theory is always based upon more than a comparison of that theory with the world. The decision to reject one paradigm is always simultaneously the decision to accept another, and the judgment leading to that decision involves comparison of both paradigms with nature *and* with each other. [Kuhn 1970, p. 77]

There is no absolute court of appeal; there are only alternate world views with fertile basic metaphors. This book attempts to trace in some detail a process of paradigm change in metaphor from machine to organic system that took the ground out from under atomism and animism alike in developmental biology. But in the end the essay must also ask how adequate Kuhn's model truly is in this field of biology. Surely it will be possible to tell the story of twentieth-century embryology in terms of Kuhn's paradigm switch. Yet how exactly, to what depth, in how essential a way does to Kuhnian scheme apply?

So far, the fundamental objection raised against a positivist view of science and history has been that inadequate attention is given to the role of metaphor.[4] Does such an objection reduce theories of scientific knowledge and progress to a type of formal literary criticism? The question ultimately concerns the nature of language. A neutral observation language, at least as a goal, is central to positivistic assumptions. Kuhn believes that the program of operationalism makes the history of science incomprehensible and the status of a scientific theory sterile.[5] Operations and manipulations, he feels, are determined by the paradigm and nothing could be practically done in a laboratory

4. The argument to follow is directed in particular against the type of approach taken by Pierre Duhem in his 1914 book *La théorie physique*, Duhem allows a certain heuristic role to models but denies that theories are essentially embedded in models and lose their coherence and comprehensiveness when uprooted from a rich, metaphoric soil. Campbell (1920) provided the classical argument against Duhem. Campbell's view of model is compatible with the one adopted here. But it is necessary to explore the differences, if any, between physics and biology in the use of metaphoric systems.

5. Ernst Mach in *The Science of Mechanics* early stated the positivist, operationalist perspective. Theories do not say anything *new* about phenomena or their structured relationships but are economical systems for restating the content of operations. This radical empiricism has been attacked many times, for example by F. P. Ramsey, but it remains influential under various guises. Probably P. W. Bridgman's 1927 *Logic of Modern Physics* gives the best account of the program for eliminating nonoperational concepts from physics.

without one (Kuhn 1970, p. 125). A pure observation language as the basis of science exactly inverts the order of things. Operationalism might make sense as a posttheoretical exercise in clarification, but it does not help in the process of planning experiments or in judging the fit of expectation and result. Further, the theory must be "reintegrated," at least tacitly, after positivist analysis if it is to make sense, that is, for its structural character to show. The reverse of the positivist claim seems to be the case: the positivist program is the useful device but a richer conception is required to generate or understand science. As Steven Pepper (1961) observes, structural coordination and empirical and logical data are necessary for adequacy. Positivism admits only the last two elements to science. Metaphoric systems are the core of structural coherence. Kuhn feels that philosophy of science from the English-speaking world "analyzes the logical structure of a completed body of scientific knowledge (Kuhn 1962, p. 136). History is suppressed in the formalization of a particular system. The formalization does not codify a pure body of knowledge stable for all future time. The rich languages used in actual science (including any axiom systems complicated enough to generate arithmetic) embody expectations and fundamental views of the structure of nature. Scientific theories are *therefore* testable and generate crisis and subsequent change.

Mary Hesse in her *Models and Analogies in Science* (1966) gives a more complete critique of the inadequacies of positivist views of science. She discusses various efforts to avoid the basic pitfalls of pure operationalism, which include versions of the hypothetical-deductive method (dictionary theories, in her language). The basic program of positivism and its offspring has been to eliminate from science theoretical terms that lack direct, observable, empirical consequences. The stumbling block has been that success in the program would make all theories tautologies, static restatements of what is already known in a longer form in terms of direct operations and observations (Hesse 1961, p. 8). The theory would lack "growing points." Loaded terms might be another expression for theoretical concepts pregnant with "impure" expectation because of the paradigm metaphor or model in which they are embedded. Hesse gives a number of paradigm model examples from physics such as wave fronts in quantum physics (pp. 8, 17), but as many can be drawn from biology, one of the most suggestive perhaps being the gene concept. The idea of the genetic particle went far beyond what could have been operationally defined, and precisely because of that fact, it was fruitful in the development of genetics.[6]

It is now possible to explore more carefully what is meant in this essay by a metaphor with explanatory power. A metaphor is the vital spirit of a paradigm (or perhaps its basic organizing relation). Hesse sees metaphor as an intrinsic part of science because metaphor is predictive. According to the formalist view of theories, "it can never be more than a lucky accident that a satisfactory isomorphism is found" between theory and nature.[7] The number of meanings applicable to theoretical terms is indefinite and there are no systematic criteria for searching out correspondences. Science becomes too arbitrary. In the metaphoric view, testing an implied isomorphism is the normal procedure. But metaphor is not just pleasing comparison. Hesse gives a provocative analysis of the logical status of analogical explanation (1966, pp. 52–129). She sees analogy between two areas from three aspects: positive, neutral, and negative. Formalist philosophies of science restrict analogy in science to the positive points of correspondence.

Comparison of theory and analogy is then a didactic device and a posttheoretic operation. Other sorts of analogy might have been useful to the scientist but would not be an intrinsic logical part of scientific knowledge. Analogy would then have a private function only. It would not be part of public science. Hesse contrasts such formal analogy with material analogy, whose essence is the possession of causal implications.[8] A metaphor is important to the nature of explanation because it leads to the testing of the neutral parts of the analogy. It leads to a searching for the *limits* of the metaphoric system and thus generates the anomalies important in paradigm change.

An important consideration in Hesse's view is the theory given by Max Black (1962) of interaction between metaphor and system of

6. The gene also has had to become less atomistic in the process, the particle metamorphosing into a system with structural laws somewhere between 1920 and 1960, the same period that saw the development of nonvitalist organicism and structuralism in developmental biology. But, of course, that system is firmly rooted in biochemistry.

7. Hesse 1966, p.46. The terms *paradigm* and *metaphor* require further clarification. Paradigm, the wider notion, includes techniques, examples, community values, and the central metaphor. A metaphor is generally related to a sense object—such as a machine, crystal, or organism. A metaphor is an image that gives concrete coherence to even highly abstract thought.

8. Ibid., pp. 79–80. A decision on the ultimate nature of causality is not necessary to the point. The logical status of analogy is a problem no matter what view is adopted toward causality. The fundamental assertion is that scientific *knowledge* is richer than theory understood as deductive system with rules of application.

phenomena under investigation. Again one is immediately returned to the problem of the nature of language. There is no correct literal description of anything by which an analogy should be judged (Hesse 1966, p. 166). Analogy and primary referent are both altered in meaning as a result of juxtaposition. The example given by Hesse is that "nature becomes more like a machine in the mechanical philosophy, and actual, concrete machines themselves are seen as if stripped down to their essential qualities of mass in motion" (p. 163).

It is important to both Black's and Hesse's points that metaphor be seen as *intelligible,* with real impact and consequences explored by communities sharing the language and image. The point is the same as Kuhn's defense of paradigm as a community possession. Metaphor is predictive because it is embedded in a rich system not private to any one man. The conditions necessary for metaphor to be explanatory are not loose. They can be summarized as the requirements that the metaphor have neutral points of analogy to be explored, that the metaphor contain the germ of concrete expectations, and that it give definite limits to acceptable theoretical accounts in science. Metaphor is a property of language that gives boundaries to worlds and helps scientists using real languages to push against these bounds. Thus one returns to Kuhn's point that the activity of normal science, puzzle solving within a particular world, itself leads to the anomalies preceding paradigm change.

One of the principal foci of this book is what Kuhn calls the quasi-metaphysical aspects of a paradigm (1970, p. 41): the sorts of entities scientists visualize as the stuff of the universe. Descartes' immense influence was a major factor in the dominant scientific belief after the mid-seventeenth century that the universe was composed of minute corpuscles. Particular kinds of motion and interaction were part of the world picture of Cartesian atomism. The paradigm functioned like a map to the structure of things.[9] The world picture functions to exclude other perceptions. It is important to stress, however, that as a consequence of the central role of metaphor paradigms operate more as directing tendencies than as clear and tyrannical logical archetypes.

9. This essay does not deal directly with the thorny problems set for Western dualistic science by Hume and Kant. Terms such as *structure* and *isomorphism* are meant to point to a modified realism, much like that suggested by A. N. Whitehead in *Process and Reality.* The mechanistic dodge of salvaging empiricism and positivism by dealing with the world only *as if* it were made of atoms will be treated later.

Kuhn treats operation of the paradigm as analogous to the *gestalt* of psychology. However, in science one does not have the option of switching perceptions back and forth, and the community of working scientists is not always aware that its vision has shifted. The pedagogical methods of science systematically suppress history, and a person sees basically only his own world and its possibilities. Kuhn gives the example of Galileo's pendulum versus the Aristotelian's falling stone (1962, p. 113), but biological examples also abound. A critical one for this essay is the perception of the organism in relation to the crystal. If one sees the world in atomistic terms (metaphysically and methodologically), the crystal is a smaller, simpler version of the organism in a nearly literal sense. If one sees the world in terms of hierarchically organized levels (the organism becomes the primary metaphor), the crystal becomes an intermediate state of organization. There is no longer a continuum of forms all based on a corpuscular foundation but rather a discontinuous series of "organisms." The crystal is still a fruitful metaphor used very seriously in exploring structure. But one sees a different crystal, just as Galileo saw a pendulum not a falling stone.

Phillip Ritterbush in his essay *The Art of Organic Forms* outlines a number of suggestive approaches to the use of metaphor in biology, in particular the use of the crystal analogy (1968). Nehemiah Grew (1628–1712), an early plant anatomist, regarded regularities in natural forms as evidence that the processes of growth consisted of the repetition of simple steps, in which forms might be successfully analyzed.[10] Ritterbush notes that in the nineteenth century Ernst Haeckel, operating on a permutation of the crystal analogy combined with an idea of ideal types, analyzed the radiolarians. His drawings show animals that are "wonders of symmetry and design. Under the influence of his aspirations to discover strict symmetry, Haeckel altered his drawings to conform to his belief in the geometrical character of organic form" (Ritterbush 1968, p. 64). Bütschli (1848–1920), still influenced by the crystal metaphor, analyzed protoplasm in terms of a geometrical space-lattice. Belief in his paradigm led to his seeing structures that could hardly be confirmed today. This fact does not belittle Bütschli's contribution to cell biology but points out the importance of his aesthetic predispositions and the power of a metaphor (p. 67). Thomas Huxley, an untainted empiricist in philosophy, nonetheless made a major

10. Ritterbush 1968, p. 8. See also Grew 1965.

advance in the classification of coelenterates by modifying an ideal
body plan to explain the place of a whole group of difficult organisms
(p. 56).

The illustration of the significance of aesthetic commitments in the
development of biology raises an important point. Ritterbush develops
the thesis of the progressive concretization of the idea of organic form.
In contrast to the atomistic analysis of the form of organisms, Goethe
(1749–1832) stated clearly and powerfully the concept of organic form.
Goethe is not considered primarily a biologist, but his impact on the
development of that science is significant.[11] Ritterbush's provocative
thesis is that biology can be seen as a concretization of an initial aesthetic notion. The metaphor of organic form became progressively more
powerful as it became more concrete, never losing its nature as metaphor. A perfect instance of the thesis is the elaboration of the cell theory
in the nineteenth century. The sphere had long been regarded as a
perfect form, appropriate to organic nature in contrast to crystalline
units. Schleiden went beyond the opposition of the two notions in a
great synthetic step, seeing the globular units of organisms as a fundamental structural basis.

> The cell theory provided a representation of the whole organism
> as an assembly of essentially similar structural units which always
> arose from pre-existing cells. This was a scientific representation
> because it referred to structure and function but also because it
> precisely fulfilled the esthetic requirements of the idea of organic
> form. In the development of the cell theory we witness the trans-
> formation of esthetic presuppositions into scientific knowledge in a
> manner that parallels Kant's statement that the sense of beauty
> is an aid to the discovery of truth.[12]

11. A useful discussion of the relation of Goethe's scientific theories to his poetry is to be found in
Salm 1971.

12. Ritterbush, 1968, pp. 33–34. The establishment of the cell theory also meant the triumph of
atomism in nineteenth-century biology. But the cell theory has been transformed in an organismic
paradigm and fills a different role. Development of the cell theory was an important nodal point in
the history of the mechanist–vitalist controversy. The crisis in embryology rooted in the Roux–
Driesch experiments of the late nineteenth century and resulting in a nonvitalist organicism in developmental biology must be seen in a nuanced and complex historical context. The debate
between Mueller and Schwann was only partly over the former's avowed vitalism. The basic disagreement hinged on the relation of part to whole, the issue that is also central to the later embryological debates. Mueller insisted that the nature of each part is influenced by its relation to the
whole; Schwann sought causes only at the level of the smallest organic elements (see Schwann
1847 and Mueller 1839).

Ritterbush sees the reduction of ideal form to objective knowledge of biological structure as a fundamental paradigm that makes the "process of biology a coherent sequence from the cell theory to DNA" (p. 34). The paradigm of the objectification of organic form is not identical to the organismic paradigm that became explicit in this century. Nevertheless, the two are closely linked and both have been important in transforming our notions of the structure–function dichotomy in science in general

Several workers of late nineteenth- and early twentieth-century biology are important from the perspective of both paradigms. For example, the German embryologist Hans Driesch was instrumental in breaking the limits of a too simple mechanism in biology and in precipitating the crisis leading to a nonvitalist organicism. But he violated the mandate of the concretization paradigm in postulating an entelechy as the director of developing form. He relapsed into the ideal, and if anything, weakened the aesthetic appeal of his explanations. D'Arcy Wentworth Thompson (1860–1948), British biologist and classical scholar, also is relevant to both paradigms. In his treatment of the theory of transformations, he illuminates the geometrical relationships that exist between closely related species. Treating the transformation of fields as a whole, he concretized the notion of type and also applied systematic criteria (1917).

The focus of this study is a period of crisis and reformulation of basic concepts in experimental embryology and cell biology. The two major concepts sketched above, that of the significance of metaphor in a revolutionary change of paradigm and that of the progressive concretization of aesthetic dictates, together form the core of the analysis. Three principal scientific workers have been chosen for careful consideration: Ross G. Harrison, Joseph Needham, and Paul Weiss. Ross Harrison (1870–1959) was a pioneer in the construction of a modern organicism in distinction to the old vitalisms and mechanisms. Trained at Johns Hopkins with W. K. Brooks and at the University of Bonn with Moritz Nussbaum, Harrison brought experimental embryology to Yale in 1907, where he remained until his death. His extraordinarily rich scientific career included development of tissue culture, a technique that he used to demonstrate the nature of nerve outgrowth (1917b). His major work was an analysis of the establishment of the axes of symmetry in the developing limb bud and inner ear of the newt. His keen interest in problems of pattern and symmetry led him to one of the most beautiful experimental treatments of form problems on the "biological level" ever undertaken. Harrison's experimental work and perceptive analysis of its implications establish him as a primary foundation stone in the edifice of molecular biology, especially as molecular study is concerned with problems of function, structure, and integration of wholes and complex systems. Harrison's work spans the years of crisis in developmental biology in the first quarter of the twentieth century and terminates as the new paradigm was becoming firmly established in the 1930s and 1940s. His work was rooted in the fertile mechanistic school of *Entwicklungsmechanik* (developmental mechanics) and developed into a mature tree transcending the old metaphors and programs. Harrison's work on the limb bud helped lay the foundation for the controversial field concept that informed so much biological work in the 1930s. The concept of the field, considerably modified since the 1930s, still supports the organismic paradigm today. Also, Harrison's associations with Hans Spemann, the German worker on the "organizer" in amphibian development, and with Paul Weiss illustrate the role of paradigm communities sketched by Kuhn. From the perspectives of the transformation of the mechanistic crystal analogy to apply to hierarchies and fields, of participation in pivotal paradigm communities, and of his central concern with the form problem in development, Harrison stands as a critical figure for a nonvitalist, experimental approach to modern organismic frameworks. Yet Harrison also is refractory to analysis in terms of paradigm revolution; he is a subtle blend of the old and the new, the continuous and the discontinuous.

Joseph Needham (b. 1900), a student of the father of British biochemistry at Cambridge, F. G. Hopkins, saw as his major scientific task the union of the areas of biochemistry and morphogenesis. He viewed both fields as absolutely essential to a proper understanding of the central problem of developmental biology, that of form and pattern. Following the discovery by Hilde Mangold and Hans Spemann in the 1920s that a piece of the dorsal lip of the amphibian blastopore implanted in the blastocoele of another embryo so as to be in contact with ventral ectoderm results in the formation of an organized secondary embryo, Needham worked with C. H. Waddington and Dorothy Needham on the chemical nature of the "organizer." He remained convinced that structure and function, form and chemical composition, were inseparable and could be dealt with experimentally without the old dichotomies. Even though the original problem of the organizer

and induction remains unsolved and even ignored, his vision has been
vindicated many times over in the concerns and achievements of
modern developmental biology. Needham was a Christian socialist
impressed with the logic and philosophy of dialectical materialism as an
alternative to the static systems of mechanism and vitalism. He was also
influenced by the organic mechanism of Alfred North Whitehead and
perceived that the revolutionary developments in physics and psychology in this century were pregnant with significance for the guiding
principles of biology. Organization and organism became the dominant
themes of his work. Needham provided one of the first full statements
of the organismic paradigm.

Beginning with World War II and a position in Chungking as liaison
between Chinese and British scientists, Needham's major interests
shifted to the history of Chinese science and technology. He abandoned
direct experimental work in the early 1940s to pursue his historical
questions. Thus the period of interest for this thesis extends from Needham's dissertation work in 1925 on the metabolic behavior of inisotol
in the developing avian egg to his insightful publications with A. S. C.
Lawrence and Shih-Chang Shen in 1944 on the anomalous viscosity
and flow birefringence of protein solutions taken from embryonic
tissues at critical points in development (Lawrence, Needham, and
Shih-Chang). From the beginning of his scientific life, Needham was
acutely interested in the philosophical and historical dimensions of
science. His writings up to the early 1930s on mechanism and vitalism,
culminating in the important Terry Lectures of 1932 (1936), are a
valuable record of the nature of the controversies of that period. He
has continued since that time to publish papers on the philosophical
status of organicism, one of the most interesting being his study (1943)
of the significance of Whitehead for biology written in 1941. He has
also continued to note in provocative papers the progress of his old
direct scientific interest, the chemical nature and specificity of the
organizer (1968). The problem is indispensable for a full understanding
of the ties between chemistry and morphogenesis.

If Harrison pioneered in laying the ground work for a biological
organicism and Needham explicitly stated the implication of the paradigm, Paul Weiss (b. 1898) has spent a life time constructing a full
organismic conception of biology and the organism. Weiss, born and
educated in Vienna, studied both engineering and the life sciences. He
brought the systems concepts of engineering to the problems posed by

the developing embryo (1925b). Drawing on the fertile analogy from physics, Weiss developed the field concept for developmental biology (1925). His early work on the regeneration of limbs led him to the concept of "resonance," highlighting a system of interaction between peripheral and central nervous structure and function. He has worked on problems of nerve growth, pattern of outgrowth under various conditions in tissue culture, organ formation as a cooperative product of cell and cell matrix interaction, neuroplasmic flow in nerves, and numerous other fundamental problems of morphogenesis and function. His experimental work on cell shape and movement and interaction has been constantly informed by an appreciation of the organism as a system-whole. Weiss exemplifies the biologist who takes organization as his basic problem, rather than as a verbal solution to profound questions.

Weiss, like Needham and Harrison, is instructive on the nature of paradigm communities. His connections with the work and thought of Harrison date from before his 1930 work at Yale. He currently participates in a community of scientists, the Alpbach group, from several fields working out organismic or structural paradigms. Needham's connection with the Theoretical Biology Club has already been mentioned. C. H. Waddington, a member of that fascinating group of the 1930s and co-worker with Joseph Needham on the chemical nature of the organizer, took part in the Alpbach Symposium with Weiss. Waddington, with his concepts of genes and pattern and of chreods, or structured pathways in development, perhaps more than anyone else has built the foundation for viewing developmental biology as a structuralism related philosophically to the psychology of Piaget and anthropology of Levi-Strauss. The organismic paradigm with its associated metaphors has permeated the heart of modern science (Piaget 1967a, 1967b).

Harrison, Needham, and Weiss also demonstrate the role of aesthetic factors in suggesting experimental work and directing its interpretation. Weiss has explicitly analyzed the relation of art and science in a provocative later article, "Beauty and the beast" (1955). Our study will look carefully at the progressive concretization of aesthetic notions resulting from the thought of all three men.

It is possible at this point to be more explicit about the questions and plan of the book. Is it legitimate to hold that a major new paradigm developed for embryology in the 1920s and 1930s? If so, what are the fruitful metaphors and models and how do they differ from the key images of the previous period? What is the nature of the crisis generated by the normal science preceding the postulated revolution? How do the new paradigm communities develop and function? What are the weaknesses of the paradigm notion for embryology? Finally, what is the relation of the organismic paradigm in biology to developments in other sciences? It is possible to maintain that branches of physics, mathematics, linguistics, psychology, and anthropology have all experienced revolutionary and related changes in dominant philosophical perspective. The primary element of the revolution seems to be an effort to deal with systems and their transformations in time; that is, to take both structure and history seriously without reducing wholes to least common denominators. Organization and process become the key concerns rather than last ditch incantations.

But before looking directly at the work and intellectual allegiances of Harrison, Needham, and Weiss, it is necessary to analyze the nature of the mechanism–vitalism controversy in order to put it in historical context. The next section looks at the years from about 1850 to 1930 as years of crisis in biology. Theories of tropisms, physiology, biochemistry, developmental mechanics—all illustrate both the triumphs of work conducted under the mechanistic program and the strains leading to the new paradigm. The major long-standing dualities in biology—structure–function, epigenesis–preformation, form–process—have all been reformulated as a result of the crisis. The section following the historical survey deals with four basic elements of the organismic paradigm. First is the primacy of the form problem, then the roles of symmetry, polarity, and pattern concepts in the old and new metaphoric systems. Third, the nature of the fiield–particle duality is examined with emphasis on the resolution offered by a nonvitalist organicism. Finally, the relationship of organicism in biology to structuralism as a philosophy is considered with the focus on the fundamental concept of organizing relationships. The following three parts of the book consider in detail the work of Harrison, Needham, and Weiss. The conclusion evaluates the adequacy of the paradigm idea in discussing change in biology and finally differentiates among Harrison, Needham, and Weiss in their degree of adherence to the organismic paradigm.

Brief Historical Sketch

In 1850 Wilhelm Roux was born in Germany. Setting up a program

and a method for the experimental analysis of development within
a mechanistic world, he was to see himself as the Descartes of
embryology.[13] But before considering his program and its effects on
embryology, it is necessary to look at the long and complicated interaction of mechanism and vitalism. In this way it will be possible to understand of significance of Roux's school of Entwicklungsmechanik.

Joseph Needham in his article "Hunting of the Phoenix" sketches
the oscillations of mechanism and vitalism in biology (1931a).[14] His
version of the history has been chosen to emphasize his conception of
revolutionary change in his own work. In a curious sense Paracelsus in
the sixteenth century is the father of both the vitalistic and mechanistic
modulations of the machine theme. He gave birth to modern chemistry
through the school of iatrochemists that followed him. But side by side
with his views on "chymical medicines" was his development of the role
of "archaei," or spirits, as governors of the chemical processes. The
fundamental ambivalence of Paracelsus was prophetic for the historical
and logical development of the mechanism–vitalism controversy.

The seventeenth century saw the full flowering of the mechanical
corpuscular philosophy. This was Whitehead's "century of genius,"
producing Newton, Leibnitz, Descartes, Harvey, Boyle, Galileo,
Francis Bacon, Pascal, Locke. On and on the list grows, including
virtually all the names a liberally educated person would recognize in
the history and philosophy of science until the mind-shaking developments in contemporary science. There is good reason these are the
names remembered, for the seventeenth century articulated and en-
throned the paradigm and its metaphoric system, which reigned until
this century. In Kuhn's terms, and consonant with Needham's views,
the intervening 200 years were a time of puzzle solving. The core of the
paradigm was summed up by Robert Boyle, author of the *Sceptical
Chemist* of 1680, "I do not expect to see any principles propos'd more
comprehensive and intelligible than the Corpuscularian or Mechanical." The seventeenth century gave science a method, a metaphysic,
and a coherent fabric of expectation that was forcibly exploited in the
following centuries. It is difficult to choose a single man from that cen-

13. Jane M. Oppenheimer drew this analogy in a conversation on July 20, 1970.

14. Much of the analysis that follows is seriously oversimplified. Mechanism and vitalism have
developed in biology since the earliest recorded observations of the Greeks, but I feel that the
simplification is legitimate in highlighting the particular crisis of the late nineteenth and early
twentieth centuries. For a recent useful summary of the period, see Coleman 1971.

tury as the most influential, but surely René Descartes would be hard to pass over. He is instructive too for the current of ambivalence in mechanism that expressed itself in various vitalistic reactions. Descartes clearly provided for a transcendent principle to plan and service his machine. His dualism was complete, and his mechanic was as necessary logically as his animal–machine. (Descartes 1955). When his successors tried to banish the substance of mind and to construct a monism of mechanical materialism, the ghost in the machine reappeared just often enough to spook the factory workers and technicians.[15] No arguments of logic would banish the vitalists, because the issue was essentially not a logical one. The metaphor and its rationale led to a vitalism as surely as it led to a mechanism. The mechanists continually embarrassed the vitalists by solving difficult puzzles on mechanical principles, and the attitudes of the vitalists often enough made their suspect status well earned. But the splits of mind and body, structure and function, efficient and final cause were never sutured during the reign of corpuscular philosophy.

The late seventeenth century saw a wave of reaction to rigid mechanism in the *anima sensitiva* of the chemist–physiologist Georg Ernst Stahl. But the eighteenth century was again dominated by discrete bits of matter in blind motion. Vitalists in this context often had a richer view of the organism. *Man a Machine* by Julien de la Mettrie, physician of the Enlightenment monarch Frederick the Great, was an expression of full, naive materialism applied to the workings of the finest timepiece of all, the human body. It is ironic that current excitement with timing and rhythm in nature might owe a great deal to the mechanical clock metaphor of Enlightenment science. If anything, the anonymous answer *Man more than a Machine* only served to emphasize the strength of the machine paradigm. The pair of articles from the eighteenth century provided the images and inspiration for Needham's *Man a Machine* written in 1928, in which he sums up his neomechanism of those years (1928a). His own realization of the implications of the new organicism dawned gradually.

The nineteenth century was to witness the triumph of mechanistic explanation in biology but also ironically the birth of the strains that were to contribute to a major crisis. Yet the strains are not so surprising

15. Koestler 1967. It is instructive to note that Koestler is a friend of Paul Weiss and was the organizer of the Alpbach Symposium. However, Koestler's and Waddington's views differ significantly, especially on genetics.

from Kuhn's perspective of normal science generating its own contradictions for the new synthesis. Needham singles out two important developments of the century as critical to the power and acceptance of mechanism: the synthesis of urea, an organic molecule, by purely chemical means by Wöhler in 1828 and the demonstration by Atwater and Rosa in 1897 that the law of conservation of energy applies strictly to animal metabolism.[16] Also, by 1840 explicit atomism had been triumphantly established in biology by the cell theory. Dalton's atom did the same for chemistry. By 1859 Darwin had published his *Origin of Species*, a work that was in many ways suspect to the archmechanists of biology (Sachs, Loeb, and Roux). But the *Origin* represented a kind of thinking very compatible with the corpuscular world view. Natural selection was not unlike the invisible hand of Adam Smith. The free play of forces and the lack of internal constraints and organizing relations were central. The Enlightenment's ideal of untrammeled reason, progress, and materialism was pervasive in the biological as well as in the social order of things.

It is instructive to look at the situation in Germany in the mid-nineteenth century, for it will be in a German context that the neovitalist Driesch will pose a fundamental challenge at the end of the century to Roux's Cartesian prophecy for embryology. The Mechanistic Quadrumvirate of Helmholtz, Ludwig, Du Bois-Reymond, and Brücke swore a mutual oath in 1845 to explain all bodily processes in mechanistic terms. This group did not make its mechanism a final metaphysic and tolerated various philosophical stances outside biology. But the step from method to metaphysic is an easy one. The medical materialists of the 1850s took the step in no uncertain terms. Jacob Moleschott, Ludwig Büchner, and Carl Vogt are "remembered for their outrageous dicta that man is what he eats, genius is a question of phosphorus, and the brain secretes thought as the kidney secretes urine."[17] At about the

16. "Hunting of the Phoenix," in 1931a, p.115. However, full application of the law of conservation of energy to animals had actually been demonstrated by Max Rubner in 1893. The essential content of the law was already widely accepted, and Rubner felt compelled to justify his extensive efforts (1894). Also, the synthesis of urea did not have the critical effect Needham ascribed to it, having more to do with the perplexity over the intricacies of organic catalysis than with the distinction between vitalists and mechanists. Liebig interpreted Wöhler's discovery in terms of a clear separation of catalytic and vital processes (see Samuel 1972). Origin of form, not chemical composition, was the real issue for vitalism and mechanism (see Brooke 1968).

17. Loeb 1964. The quote is from Fleming's introduction, p. ix. For a discussion of important issues in physiology and biochemistry relevant to this dissertation, see the introduction by Frederic L. Holmes to Justus Liebig's *Animal Chemistry* (1964). See also Galaty (1974), for a discussion of the philosophical basis of mid-nineteenth century reductionism.

same time, Rudolf Virchow, the celebrated physiologist, published "The mechanistic conception of life."[18]

It was in this atmosphere that Jacques Loeb (1859–1924) developed. Tormented by a deep need to resolve the issue of free will and determinism in human action, Loeb found a solution in his doctrine of animal tropisms, first elaborated about 1880. He was a student of the plant physiologist, Julius Sachs, at the University of Würzburg. Another of Loeb's teachers, Adolf Fick, had been in his turn a student of Ludwig and Du Bois-Reymond of the Mechanistic Quadrumvirate. Sachs developed the concept of plant tropisms.[19] Loeb became the apostle of the significance of the new physical chemistry for explanation in biology. The important contemporary experiments of Arrhenius on electrolysis were vital to his own work on osmotic phenomena in animals. The power of Loeb's approach is important as an illustration of the high tide of mechanism in biology.[20]

In 1911 in Hamburg at the First International Congress of Monists, convened by Ernst Haeckel, Loeb gave a speech printed in the following year as *The Mechanistic Conception of Life*. In that address Loeb outlined his theory of tropisms. It is interesting that in the body of the talk he

18. J. S. Haldane's opinions later in the century on the secretion of oxygen by lung tissue made him a vitalist; it is amusing to speculate what his opponents would have thought had he proposed that the brain secretes thought. Even modern membrane physiologists would hesitate to postulate the precise mechanism of such active transport. It might be noted too that Feuerbach held opinions similar to the medical materialists on the nature of man and nutrition.

Virchow and the medical materialists related their scientific doctrines directly to their radical socialism in opposition to the Prussian state. An important chapter in the history of science must be concerned with the relation between social and scientific commitments. It has been noted that Needham, a socialist, was an influential organicist who was explicit about using dialectical materialism *in* science. Gary Werskey, lecturer at the Science Studies Unit of the University of Edinburgh, has written a provocative dissertation about the important British socialist scientists of the 1930s, J. D. Bernal, L. Hogben, Needham, J. B. S. Haldane, and others.

19. A tropism is an obligatory movement made by an organism in a response directly proportional to a physical stimulus such as light or gravity. The debt of Loeb to Sachs is only one example of the close relation of botany to the development of embryology. Ross Harrison was deeply indebted to both Sachs and Gottlieb Haberlandt, who first tried to culture the cells of higher plants. Jane Oppenheimer also makes a strong argument that Harrison was influenced early by Hermann Vöchting, an investigator of plant polarity (see Oppenheimer 1967, p. 110). Harrison's lifelong associate, Sally Wilens, feels there is insufficient evidence in the Harrison papers for Vöchting's influence.

20. In this essay oversimplified examples from physiology have been incorporated for several reasons. Mechanism was historically more fruitful for physiology than for embryology. Jacques Loeb forms one link between the two sciences. Also, the physiologist J. S. Haldane was important to Needham's judgments on mechanism and vitalism. Finally, Wilhelm Roux saw himself applying the powerful tools developed in a mechanistic framework, long well-exploited in physiology, to the problems of embryology.

never states precisely *which* organisms he means when he says that
"animals" respond in a certain way to light. The animal machine was
a powerful abstraction.[21] He worked on the coelenterate *Eudendrium*
and the marine worm *Spirographis*, showing that they turn to light just
as positively heliotropic plants do. Such determinisms underlie even
the most complex phenomena, including those of that other great
abstract entity, the "will."

A second aspect of Loeb's work more directly relevant to embryology
is his investigation of artificial fertilization and parthenogenesis.
Flemming states that the demonstration of the possibility of raising
healthy sea urchin larvae without participation by the sperm "was
the feat that captured the imagination of the world" (Loeb 1964,
p. xxiii). Physical factors alone could trigger all the complex processes
of development.

Work proceeding from the concept of tropisms generated the contradictions and strains that were to contribute to the approaching crisis
of mechanism. By 1894 C. Lloyd Morgan in England had developed
the concept of trial and error in animal learning. It was H. S. Jennings,
an American student of animal behavior and author of several papers
on mechanism and vitalism in biology, who used the concept of trial
and error against Loeb's conception of tropism. Jennings believed that
his work flowed from Loeb's lead in the objective analysis of behavior.
Yet in 1906 Jennings demonstrated that many lower organisms did
not display true tropistic behavior but rather showed spontaneous
activities until a chance course of action relieved distress. Pure determinism did not explain even the behavior of simple animals. Jennings's
work hardly toppled mechanism, and he rejected all vitalism vigorously
(Loeb 1964, p. xxxvii). But the refractory nature of animal behavior
to inclusion in the pure machine paradigm was an important backdrop
in the development of organicism.

Before organicism was born, many outstanding biologists went

21. Loeb 1964, p. 29. The identification Loeb actually gives is, "I found the same phenomenon,
i.e. positive heliotropism, in sessile animals, *e.g.* certain hydroids and worms." In another section of
the paper he discusses similar experiments on a beast with eyes and muscles and the power of movement in response to light. In no place in the paper from the speech or its illustrations is the animal
identified even as to phylum. The point to be made is similar to the famous one made by Whitehead
in reference to mechanistic physics. To consider simple location as the fundamental reality is not
"wrong," it is a case of misplaced concreteness. Loeb expresses the tremendous abstract nature of
his creed; the paradigm of progressive concretization of the conceptions of animal form and process
suffers.

through a stage of neovitalism. Needham felt that three workers in particular had deserted the straight and narrow and had invited the demon back into the machine oiled and put in running order by the energetic craftsmen of mechanism: J. S. Haldane, E. S. Russell, and Hans Driesch. Haldane was a physiologist, Russell a student of animal behavior, and Driesch an embryologist. Biology owes to all three a great deal of fundamental work. None of the three judged mechanist analysis adequate to explain the phenomena he dealt with daily. Haldane, who with J. G. Priestly did a basic analysis of animal respiration (1935), developed the idea of "nostalgia." He emphasized the wholeness of the organism and the inadequacy of mechanism to account for purposeful behavior and, specifically, for the unity of the life history of the organism (Haldane 1931). His nostalgia was perhaps analogous to the *conatus* of Spinoza. The charge of vitalism is difficult to maintain against Haldane, but it is certain he was struggling through a period of dissatisfaction with the metaphors and explanatory power of the machine paradigm. But he did not formulate a clear, alternative organicism. As Needham observed, Haldane tended to let the word *organization* take the place of a definite program of experiment and intellectual framework (1932, p. 110).

Russell, in attempting to bridge the mind–body split of post-Cartesian science, emphasized the directive character of organic life. His mistake came in seeing direction in terms of a future state of the organism instead of in terms of the present configuration of the whole system. This perspective was classically Aristotelian. The nonvitalist organicists, although deeply indebted to Aristotle, insisted that form had to be explained via process, not the reverse. Russell had no system of transformations for complex wholes, but again his service was in refusing to cover up strains in mechanism with naïve abstractions. The metaphor of the machine was unsatisfactory. The alternative appeared to be either vitalist or nebulous (Russell 1945).

Hans Driesch is the most important neovitalist for the purposes of this work. Operating from strict mechanistic expectations and under the influence of Roux, he was driven to construct an elaborate mechanic for the embryo, a reemergence of Aristotle's entelechy. But to give greater depth to the theories of Driesch and the program of Roux, it would be helpful to look again at the significance of physics and psychology for biological explanations and at the logic of the machine paradigm.

Two critical periods in the development of physics for explanatory principles in biology are obvious. The first is the seventeenth century, which witnessed the appearance of Newton's *Principia* in 1687. The essentials of the corpuscular and mechanistic philosophy were a distinction between primary and secondary qualities and a reliance on an associationist empiricism in epistemological questions. Causal analysis was the method of success, and the unity of science rested on the hope of reducing all explantions devised to deal with phenomena in the natural world to the fundamental principles of mechanics (laws of matter in motion). It is a truism to note that biology felt itself a secondary science, one sadly behind sophisticated physics. The program of Roux to begin full causal, physical, and mathematical explanation for embryology was an expression of both his confidence in the machine paradigm and his sense of the inferiority of the previous approaches of biology. If the machine analogy were not held to apply rigorously, at least explanation had to be "physical–chemical." As was evidenced by Clerk Maxwell's development of electromagnetic theory in the nineteenth century and even by the scandal of Newton's gravity, physics itself was not totally contained with in the strict machine analogy. But the assumption ran strong that the basic principles necessary for real science were all in; to say that explanation must be in physical–chemical terms but not necessarily reduced to one branch of physics, mechanics, was a slight modification. Physics and chemistry were throughly mechanistic, in hope if not fact.

Then the certainties of physics shattered in the twentieth century. In 1925 Alfred North Whitehead published his *Science and the Modern World*, in which he outlines the events of the second critical period for biology. If field theories alone had not, relativity theory and then quantum mechanics had broken the axis of the machine analogy for physics. Even the ultimate elementary unit of matter, perfectly describable by the device of primary qualities, was doing unexpected things and directing trusted, intelligent men such as Whitehead, a mathematical physicist, to think in terms of organization, wholes, and internal relations. Reductionism no longer seemed simple, because physics and chemistry themselves were outgrowing the mechanism that made this form of reductionism so attractive. The foundation for the unity of science would have to be sought elsewhere.

All these observations are very simpleminded. However, it is necessary to remember that biology could not have developed a respectable organicism until rigid determinism broke down in physics and minds were freed to feel the strains and contradictions of naïve mechanism. For anyone in the eighteenth century to have felt that biology might be more fundamental (not just blessed with *archaei*, which is cheating) than physics would have been absurd. But that is exactly what J. S. Haldane thought in the late nineteenth and early twentieth centuries. He was accused of being a vitalist; he was only a bit unclear. But Whitehead too insisted that the unity of science was based on organic "events" rather than simple atoms; he was some what clearer. C. F. A. Pantin's recent treatment of restricted (physics and chemistry) and unrestricted (biology and geology) sciences is a full flowering of the directions made possible by 1925.[22] As Kuhn noted, a crisis in a paradigm could not lead to abandonment of the paradigm until an alternative was available. Biology could not seriously explore an organicism in response to its own crises until its relation to physics was changed.[23]

22. 1968, p.24.
"In fact, the relations of the sciences is that of a multidimensional network with cross relations, as illustrated by geology and biophysics. ... One can see a general decrease in complexity as one passes from geology or biology to physics, though the complexity is not of the same kind in all the complex sciences. The simplicity of the physical sciences, combined with the attention given to them because of their immediate powerful technical consequences, is the cause of their rapid success. Intellectually magnificent though the attack on them has been, the problems they present are easier than those of the geological and biological sciences.

"There is one real, and graded, distinction between sciences like the biologies and the physical sciences. The former are *unrestricted* sciences and their investigator must be prepared to follow their problems into any other science whatsoever. The physical sciences, as they are understood, are restricted in the field of phenomena to which they are devoted. They do not require the investigator to traverse all other sciences. But while this restriction is the basis of their success, because of the introduction of this restricted simplicity of their field we cannot necessarily take them or their methods as typical of all the sciences."

23. Developments in psychology have closely paralleled those in physics. The associationist, empirical tradition from Locke and Hume gave an analysis of perception appropriate to a dualistic, mechanistic physical science. The development of Gestalt thinking and field analogies by Wolfgang Köhler in psychology in this century is important to organismic thinking in biology. Also, the revolt against the tenets of reflex theories by men such as Kurt Goldstein and then by Merleau-Ponty, who owes a large debt to Goldstein, is illustrative of the relationships among types of thinking simultaneously emerging in physics, biology, and psychology in the first quarter of the century. Perception itself comes to be seen as an organized event or whole, and traditional subject–object splits come to be seen as inappropriate approaches to psychological phenomena. Perhaps Michael Polanyi, in his *Personal Knowledge* and *Tacit Dimension*, comes closest among contemporary thinkers to an adequate theory of knowledge for an organismic biology. Of exceptional importance for understanding the structure of thought in apparently diverse but contemporary fields is Michel Foucault's *The Order of Things* (1970).

Let us look more closely at the characteristics of the machine paradigm as it was adopted in biology. The Austrian systems biologist
Ludwig von Bertalanffy wrote a book called *Kritische Theorie der
Formbildung* that appeared in English (translated by J. H. Woodger)
in 1933 with the title *Modern Theories of Development*. From the perspective of his own organicism, Bertalanffy sketched the essence of the
mechanistic–vitalistic position in developmental biology in the early
twentieth century. At least two meanings of mechanism have to be
distinguished. The first meaning is that biological laws must ultimately
be expressed in physical–chemical terms; this position is reductionism
in the sense that physics is the foundation of science. Nothing is directly
said about the nature of physical–chemical theory to which biological
explanation must be reduced. It is obviously futile to argue against
the prediction that a future body of theory will or will not comprehend
a given set of phenomena. As Whitehead observed early, physics itself
now has vastly different conceptions of organization, causality, and
determinism and thus of fundamental explanation. When the very
categories of explanation being contested are abandoned, reductionism
becomes simply a false issue.[24]

The second meaning of mechanism might be less crucial than the
controversy over reductionism to logical problems in the philosophy of
science, but it is probably more relevant historically for early twentieth-
century embryology. This form of mechanism states that the organism
is a machine and its operation can be explained by the principles of
mechanics. The issue of machine design is not considered directly any
more than the issue of mind is handled satisfactorily by a materialistic
monism that is ultimately rooted in Cartesian distinctions.[25] But just

24. Of modern philosophers of science Ernest Nagel has dealt most extensively with reductionism and claims of biology to autonomy. He remarks that it is illegitimate to deny *in principle* the
reduction of biology to physics and chemistry simply because present physical–chemical theory is
inadequate for the reduction. However, Nagel does not give sufficient attention to the nature of the
organismic paradigm. If physics and chemistry must deal with concepts of structure, regulation,
field, organization, hierarchy, and history, it is originally biological concepts that become most
basic. But in fact, nothing is being reduced, and Pantin's distinction of restricted–unrestricted
science is much more fruitful (see Nagel 1951).
25. Michael Polanyi treats the problems of machine design in a particularly creative way. The
essential notion is that of boundary conditions, a concept critical to any structuralism. Machines
and organisms both work on higher principles than those of physics and chemistry; both are
hierarchical systems of dual control. A higher level imposes boundaries on a system with degrees of
freedom left by operations of the lower level. "Hence the existence of dual control in machines and
living mechanisms represents a discontinuity between machines and living things on the one hand

as materialisms are counterbalanced by elaborate idealisms, reliance
on the machine analogy itself elicits various vitalisms. The suggestiveness of a particular metaphor is the central aspect of the old machine
theory in biology.[26]

The character of the analogy is based on certain fundamental points.
The most critical assumption can be labeled the "additive point of
view." Bertalanffy describes the perspective as follows:

> Chemistry analyses bodies into simple constituents, modecules,
> atoms, electrons; the physicist regards the storm which uproots
> the tree as the sum of the movements of all particles of air. . . . In
> the same way the physical-chemical investigation of organisms has
> consisted in the attempt to analyse them into elementary parts and
> processes. . . . The additive standpoint is expressed most clearly
> in the theory of the 'cell-state,' the attempt to resolve the living
> body into an aggregate of independent constituents, its total
> activity into cell-functions. It found its classical expressions in the
> machine theory of Weissman, in which it was assumed that the
> egg contains a collection of developmental machines for the various
> organs which unfold themselves independently of one another and
> in this way form the mature organism. In the last resort, me-
> chanism must try to resolve the action of the organism as a whole
> into *single* [emphasis added] physical-chemical processes. [1933,
> pp. 32–33]

Ernest Nagel is correct in pointing out the potential ambiguity of the
word *sum* in such passages (1951). But the principal meaning can be
described adequately. The parts of the machine are simple, unorganized, and not intrinsically altered if installed in a different place in
the mechanism. The machine probably would not work if parts were
interchanged, but even if it did one still should not talk about position
effects and true regulation. Perhaps the parts were similar enough

---

and inanimate nature on the other, so that both machines and living mechanisms are irreducible
to the laws of physics and chemistry." The relationship corresponds to Pantin's restricted–unrestricted distinction in the sciences. "Each level relies for its operation on all the levels below it.
Each reduces the scope of the one immediately below it by imposing on it a boundary that har-
nesses it to the service of the next higher level, and this control is transmitted stage by stage, down
to the basic inanimate level" (see Polanyi 1968).

26. One is not concerned here with machine in the sense of computers and self-regulating
mechanisms. Whether such machines are part of a mechanistic or organismic biology is a separate
and complicated question.

already to act in one another's roles. If regulation is an impermissible concept, one expects to find preformed parts and mosaic patterns in developmental machines (eggs and embryos). Organization then means only the configuration of preformed parts and rigid processes of the machine. The concept itself cannot be analyzed further without running into contradictions to the basic mechanistic perspective. Thus, *sum* means aggregate without additional principles or regularities specified or necessary to explain the animal–machine's operation. All "organizing relations" are external in J. H. Woodger's sense. An internal relation implies that the "parts" themselves are different depending on whether they are in or out of a particular context.[27]

Vitalism of a quasi-metaphysical kind is in opposition to mechanistic materialism as a philosophy, but it is not in opposition to the machine theory. It merely notes processes of regulation that appear in animal machines and postulates machine designers and mechanics. The machine analogy is not challenged by a wider meaning of organization or by a refusal to operate from the additive perspective.[28]

With a fuller appreciation of the nature of the machine analogy embedded in the mechanistic paradigm, it is time to look more closely at developments in embryology. The controversy that demonstrated most clearly the inadequacy of the simple machine analogy for biology centered around problems of determination and regulation in the embryo.

In the 1870s Wilhelm His attempted to turn German embryology away from its excessive formal concern with type and phylogeny. Such concerns were largely the result of the immense influence of Haeckel and his revival of *Naturphilosophie* coupled with his advocacy of Darwinism. The earlier work of Pander and von Baer had been unexploited despite its great potential for an analytical embryology. His espoused mechanical explanation for such events as the folding of the medullary plate. He met strong opposition to his approach and did not support it with a firm experimental commitment. He made so-called model experiments but did not make the decisive experiments on the living

27. Woodger 1930a (*Q. Rev. Biol.* 5:1–22).
28. Bertalanffy 1933, p.44. The most sympathetic and ample treatment of vitalism may be Johannes Mueller's in his *Element of Physiology* (1839, p. 20). 'Life, therefore, is not simply the result of the harmony and reciprocal action of these parts; but is first manifested in a principle or imponderable matter which is in action in the substance of the germ, enters into the composition of the matter of this germ, and imparts to organic combinations properties which cease at death."

organism itself. August Weismann prepared the ground for the fully experimental school of Roux with the publication in 1874 of his treatise on the germ plasm, *Das Keimplasm*. In it he developed a theory of determination based on pre-formed particles parceled out during development. Weismann's theory was a pure modern preformationism. It had a major impact on young Wilhelm Roux, who began his research into the physiology of embryological development from a central question about the extent and nature of self-differentiation. He early refuted (1885) the W. Pflüger hypothesis that gravity affected the plane of cleavage of the frog egg and concluded that the causes of bilateral symmetry must lie within the egg itself.[29] Hans Spemann notes in his Silliman Lectures of 1938 the background for Roux's famous pricking experiments on the two-cell-stage frog embryo (1938). The next question was whether those facts that had been established for the whole egg with regard to its surroundings would also hold true for all its parts with regard to one another, whether—and to what degree—their development also is self-differentiation. To answer this question, Roux excluded one part of the egg from development and tested the remaining portion for its capacity for development. Roux's famous pricking experiment exercised an enormously stimulating influence on future research (Spemann 1938, p. 18). In 1888 Roux placed a hot needle into one blastomere of the two-celled frog egg, thereby killing it (Roux 1890). He assumed that killing the cell prevented it from influencing the remaining cell.[30] The remaining cell developed into a half-embryo deficient in those parts that would normally have been contributed by the dead blastomere. This experiment led directly to Roux's mosaic theory of development. "According to this theory, all single primordia stand side by side, separate from each other, like stones of a mosaic work and develop independently, although in perfect harmony with each other, into the finished organism" (Spemann 1938, p. 20). It is impossible to miss the pointed imagery derived from the machine paradigm. The ultimate simple unit did not get involved in entangling "internal organizing relations."

29. The entire discussion on His, Weismann, Roux, and Driesch draws heavily on Oppenheimer 1967. See Churchill (1968) for further discussion of Weismann.

30. Note here the power of the mechanistic paradigm in conditioning expectations. Roux did not really expect parts to influence one another substantially. A method for completely separating amphibian blastomeres was not successful until 1895, when Endres did it for the newt egg. He got two complete small embryos. In 1910 the two blastomeres of Roux's frog egg were finally successfully separated.

Roux had set embryology on its experimental, analytical course as early as 1881 in his *Der Kampf der Theile im Organismus.*[31] The title fore-shadowed his deep interest in dependent versus independent differen-tiation. Despite Roux's mistrust of Darwinism because of Haeckel's exploitation of it in Germany, his analogy of struggle among parts was a Darwinian image. The image relies on a mechanistic paradigm wider than its use by any one worker. Roux in his autobiography of 1923 acknowledges his heavy debt to Descartes. He wanted to show that a *causalnexus* operated in embryology and that the proper method to establish causal connections was the analytical–empirical one. His paradigm was constructed within the larger framework of mechanism in physics and provided a program for research that was hardly to be soon exhausted.[32] The prolific school of Entwicklungsmechanik in-spired men such as Spemann, Harrison, and Holtfreter, an impressive list of embryologists. But the paradigm was soon to show the strains that would undermine its basic assumptions. Even all three of the above men contributed significantly to the articulation of an organicism having nothing to do with traditional vitalism and transcending Roux's machine perspective.

Expecting only to confirm the previous results of Roux on the frog egg, in 1891 Hans Driesch performed his famous experiments of separa-ting the first two blastomeres of the sea urchin egg. He dramatically describes his expectations in his Gifford Lectures of 1908 (1929). He shook the sea urchin egg until the connections between the two cells were severed. Each cell, instead of developing into a good half-embryo, formed a perfect but small complete embryo. Driesch's words are worth

31. The complete title in English is *The struggle of parts in the organism. A contribution towards the completion of a mechanical theory of teleology.*

32. Roux did not feel that all biological explanation had to be in exclusively physical–chemical terms immediately. Realization of that hope lay in the future. Investigation by analytical methods of phenomena on the biological level was appropriate and necessary in the interim. Qualitative investigation often had to precede quantitative. It is also important to note that Roux, especially in his early days, was not totally defined by his neopreformationism, mosaicism, and self-differentia-tion theories. He had a full rich set of questions for the embryo, though all those questions still acquired meaning through their relation to the machine paradigm. For example, Jane Oppenhei-mer notes Roux's work on environmental influences on the egg (1884–1891) and on the relation of developing parts to one another (1894) (see Oppenheimer 1967, pp. 66–72). These later experi-ments were on cytotropisms that influenced Holtfreter's later work (1939) on aggregation and disaggregation of cells. Roux was a friend of Jacques Loeb, advocate of animal tropisms within a mechanistic deterministic framework. Loeb, needless to add, heartily approved of Roux's program for embryology.

quoting because they show the strength of the mechanistic paradigm expectations that later throw light on his turn to the mechanic, the entelechy.

> The development of our *Echinus* proceeds rather rapidly, the cleavage being complete in about 15 hours. I quickly noticed on the evening of the first day of the experiment, when the half-embryo was composed of about two hundred cells, that the margin of the hemispherical embryo bent together a little, as if it were to form a whole sphere of smaller size, and indeed the next morning there was a whole diminutive blastula swimming about. I was so convinced that I should get the Roux effect in all its features that, even in spite of the whole blastula, I now expected that the next morning would reveal to me the half-organization of the subject once more. ... But things turned out as they were bound to do, and not as I had expected; there was a typically *whole* gastrula in my dish the next morning.[33]

The sea urchin eggs of Driesch had done what a good machine should not: they had regulated themselves to form wholes from parts. Driesch was led to develop a concept of equipotential systems in which function is dependent on position within the whole, not on any mechanical preformation of parts. Embryos for Driesch were radically indeterminate. That both Roux and Driesch were "wrong" about determination from the perspective of later work is of little importance. The battle lines were drawn. The machine paradigm had failed Driesch, but rather than abandon it, he resurrected the mechanic. His logic was impeccable, and until 1930 the embryological world occupied itself with trying to exorcise Driesch's demon. However, no spell was entirely effective until the concepts of regulation and of whole could be dealt with outside the machine paradigm. And perhaps this power is the major contribution of the new organicism to embryology.

Before turning to the work of Ross G. Harrison in an attempt to show

---

33. Needham quotes the same passage in *Order and Life* (1936, pp. 51–52) in a different context, that of discussing the roots of a topographical conception of the "deployment of biological order." Driesch introduced the concepts of prospective potency and prospective significance as a result of his experiments. Potency is greater than normal significance. As she did for Roux, Jane Oppenheimer describes for Driesch how broad his interests and work in embryology were. They extended far beyond the experiments for which the two men are remembered. Oppenheimer discusses Driesch's strong materialistic analysis in several areas of his 1894 *Analytische Theorie der organischen Entwicklung* (see Oppenheimer 1967, pp. 72–78).

how he laid the foundation for a nonvitalist organicism, it is necessary to understand clearly how we shall use four sets of concepts. They are form; symmetry, polarity, and pattern; fields and particles; and organicism as a structuralism rather than a vitalism. After some essential remarks on the history of the word *organicism*, the next section will develop the last of the raw materials for the ensuing investigation.

2

The Elements of Organicism

Moreover, when any one of the parts or structures, be it which it may, is under discussion, it must not be supposed that it is its material composition to which attention is being directed or which is the object of discussion, but the relation of such part to the total form. Similarly, the true object of architecture is not bricks, mortar, or timber, but the house; and so the principal object of natural philosophy is not the material elements, but their composition, and the totality of the form, independently of which they have no existence.

Aristotle

Ich Krystall.

Paul Klee

Is the organismic point of view a single, coherent perspective, or is the term merely a convenient cover for diverse biological doctrines? What really is the organismic paradigm? How and when did it appear in biology? Before studying the abstract elements of organicism—form; symmetry, polarity, and pattern; fields and particles—it is enlightening to review the chronological development of the term and its associated notions. All varieties of organicists trace themselves to Aristotle, especially to his intense appreciation of teleological explanation as a complement to material explanation, but recent organicists see their immediate lineage in diverse sources. Morton Beckner maintains that only in the twentieth century has it been possible to distinguish organicism as a doctrine from the varieties of vitalism (1969, pp. 549–51). Vitalism and organicism share basic questions and positions. From a negative point of view, both maintain that the study of the parts does not suffice to explain the behavior of the whole. The methods and conclusions of other sciences, in particular physics and chemistry, are held to be applicable to organisms but radically insufficient. Second,

the form of the whole is important in embryological development,
animal behavior, reproduction, and physiology. By whatever means,
the properties of the whole are as essential in determining the nature
and behavior of the parts at each stage in the life cycle as vice versa.
Last, both organicists and vitalists stress the teleological behavior of
organisms: there is at least the appearance of goal-directedness and
design in biological phenomena. These properties ensure that biology
is an autonomous science, not a postscript to physics. The idea of
autonomy will be explored in chapter 6. Nevertheless, organicists and
vitalists differ fundamentally on where they locate the root of wholeness
and consequent regulative behavior of organisms. Vitalists of all hues
assert some nonphysical entity—either a nonquantifiable vital force
like Driesch's entelechy or some basic difference between "vital substance" and ordinary matter. Organicists insist that wholeness, di-
rectedness, and regulation can be explained fully without such notions.

Several lineages have been proposed for organicism in recent biology.
The American zoologist working at the Scripps Institute in California,
W. E. Ritter, concentrates on French and American contributions to
the perspective (1919). Beckner cites Ritter as the first modern organicist, noting his introduction of the term *organismalism* to represent
the idea that "the organism in its totality is as essential to an explanation
of its elements as its elements are to an explanation of the organism."
Ritter called nature a "system" (p. x) and thought it was important
for a biologist to try to develop a general theory of natural knowledge
in order to show the integrated character of the whole world—animate,
and mental. Using the polar opposition of Aristotelian organismalism
and Lucretian elementalism, Ritter examined the history of biology
from the late eighteenth century. In turning to the great schools of
comparative anatomy in France, he found that Georges Cuvier's concept of type necessitated studying organs as parts of the whole. His
doctrine of correlations aimed at enabling the investigator to recon-
struct the whole from intimate understanding of the smallest fragment.
Geoffroy Saint-Hilaire continued the tradition in his theory of analogies, which tried to illuminate the whole through the relations of anatomical parts of diverse organisms. That Geoffroy and Cuvier considered
their own ideas and methods to be deeply opposed did not concern
Ritter.

Ritter next mentioned a group of biologists working in the first two-
thirds of the nineteenth century that included C. E. von Baer, Claude

Bernard, M. Bichât, W. His, and E. Pflüger. In his treatise *L'Hérédité* (Paris, 1903), the French author G. Delage called these workers "organicists."

Ritter attached little importance either to Delage's label or to the organicists' ideas as ancestral to his own. In fact he viewed the work of Bichât on tissues as supportive of the elementalist conception, especially as that doctrine was strengthened by the cell theory of Schwann. In Ritter's opinion, Theodor Schwann's stress on the cell as the fundamental unit of the organism underlay the regression of organismal perspectives from 1840 to 1890. In the 1890s there was a revival of the organismal point of view, but it seemed to have little to do with the work of the French anatomists of the earlier period. Rather it arose *de novo* from the consequences of the inadequacy of the elementalist approach in applying the cell theory to individual development. Ritter recognized that Roux and Driesch were testing the powers of the elemental parts. The American zoologist interpreted their results as the failure to explain ontogeny by cellular phenomena alone.

Leaving the great school of developmental mechanics at that point, Ritter turned to a group of American embryologists to make the case for the next step in the advancing organismal biology: C. O. Whitman, E. B. Wilson, and F. R. Lillie. Around the turn of the century these men critically examined the cell theory in relation to development, although none went far enough for Ritter's taste. Nevertheless, these embryologists represented the stirrings of a physiological period; that is, a study of development and correlation from the functional side, paralleling the structural organismalism of the comparative anatomists. A little later, C. M. Child's doctrine of physiological equilibrium represented significant work from the organismal point of view. In other areas of biology Starling's study of hormones and C. S. Sherrington's ideas of the nervous system extended the approach Ritter so favored.

Ritter cited but gave little attention to a book written in 1917 that sketched similar ideas but recognized different intellectual debts. The American L. J. Henderson, later important to the development of Joseph Needham's organicism through his *Fitness of the Environment* (1913), discussed the history of vitalism and mechanism in an intriguing philosophical context in *Order of Nature* (1917). Henderson maintained that the concept of organization first appeared explicitly as a problem and postulate in scientific research in the nineteenth century. The idea of organization evolved from the old notion of function in physiology. With Cuvier, organization become an explicit, conscious concept. In physiology, at least from the time of Johannes Mueller, organicism was differentiating itself from vitalism. In embryology Aristotle's old concept of internal teleology of the organism lay at the heart of von Baer's biological philosophy. Henderson, like Ritter, cited Delage's use of the term *organicist* to cover von Baer, Bichât, and later Claude Bernard. Unlike Ritter, Henderson considered Roux's school of developmental mechanics as a keystone in the experimental study of organization and integration. Ross Harrison's evolution toward organicism seems rooted both in this view of Entwicklungsmechanik and in his connection with the concerns of American embryologists such as E. B. Wilson. That Harrison, Wilson, Conklin, and other American experimental embryologists were all students of W. K. Brooks at Johns Hopkins was surely important to their shared concerns. Harrison's later, more explicit organicism was connected to Needham and Weiss through developments to be sketched in detail later. Finally, Henderson outlined the progress of the organismic approach along several independent lines: experimental morphology, physiology, and the study of metabolism. He cited such men as Roux, Sherrington, Pavlov, and Cannon. Henderson concluded with the opinion that contemporary studies of organization only translated the Aristotelian idea of internal teleology into a concrete experimental focus on self-regulation.

A second book published in 1917 but ignored by Ritter was the Englishman J. S. Haldane's *Organism and Environment*, based on a course of Silliman lectures at Yale (1917). Haldane insisted that neither vitalism nor mechanism was appropriate to the explanation of the nature of coordination of physiological activities. He is perhaps the first to choose deliberately to call himself an organicist: "It has been suggested to me that if a convenient label is needed for the doctrine upheld in these lectures the word 'organicism' might be employed. The word was formerly used in connection with the somewhat similar teaching of such men as Bichât, von Baer, and Claude Bernard. Cf G. Delage, L'Hérédité, Paris, 1903, p. 435" (p. 3). Haldane made no effort to trace a specific lineage for his views, but spent his time arguing that understanding wholeness necessitated paying attention not only to parts of the organism in relation to the total but also to the organism in relation to the environment. As pointed out in chapter 1, Joseph Needham was profoundly unimpressed by Haldane's organicism, calling it a form of neovitalism because it left words such as organization so vague.

A second Englishman is also important as an early modern organicist, E. S. Russell, another of Needham's neovitalists.[1] Without citing Ritter, Russell sketches his biological position and his opinions on intellectual ancestry in a chapter entitled "The Organismal Point of View." Like all the other organicists, he differentiated his views from both mechanism and vitalism, insisting that in particular Driesch's entelechy was useless in explaining biological organization. For Russell the notion of the organism as a unified whole could be traced in a line from Aristotle through Kant, then to the Driesch of 1912, and finally to J. S. Haldane from 1913 on. Russell saw the essence of the organismal view in its starting point: the fundamental unit of biology is the whole individual organism. Like all other organicists, Russell prefers philosophical realism. The basic objects of the natural world to which knowledge refers are given, at least as much as created for specific human intellectual or practical purposes. He traced his own ideas from what he called his methodological vitalism of 1911 through a kind of psychobiology to the positions of his 1930 book. The problem of mind and direction of animal behavior and development most occupied Russell. He believed that the views of S. Alexander, General Smuts, and C. Lloyd Morgan converged with his own. He succinctly stated the purpose of the organismal conception:

> It gives us a unitary biology, in which the abstractness and excessive analysis of the materialistic method are avoided; it allows us to look on the living thing as a functional unity, disregarding the separation of matter and mind, and to realize how all its activities—activities of the whole, and activities of the parts, right down to the intra-cellular unities—subserve in cooperation with one another the primary end of development, maintenance, and reproduction. [1930, p. 189]

So far we have seen Americans and Englishmen claim priority in

---

1. Russell 1930. The confusion over whether to label a person a vitalist or organicist will be examined in the concluding chapter. Some philosophers and historians of science claim there is little distinction. But from a Kuhnian perspective, it makes a great deal of difference whether organicism is seen as a continuation of vitalism, making the contemporary organicist–reductionist debates equivalent to the older vitalist–mechanist opposition, or whether both current labels in the debate represent fundamental changes in perspective (see Hein 1972).

developing modern organicism; each writer created his intellectual history to illuminate the significant aspects of his own thought—a typical paradigm-building practice. But still another individual was to press his paternity rights. Ludwig von Bertalanffy, who will be met yet again because of his importance for the particular organicism of Joseph Woodger and Needham, wrote that he was the first to have developed consistently the organismic perspective. Beginning in 1926, he proposed organicism, using the term explicitly in 1928 in *Kritische Theorie der Formbildung*, as an alternative to mechanism and vitalism (1952).[2] For Bertalanffy organicism was necessary to accomplish three specific jobs in biology: appreciation of wholeness (regulation), organization (hierarchy and the laws proper to each level), and dynamics (process; later, behavior of open systems). After asserting his own originality, Bertalanffy listed others he felt were working along organismic lines; the large number in diverse fields was evidence of the importance of the intellectual transformation. He cited Ritter and Russell but gave references from 1928 for Ritter, not 1919.

At least three and perhaps four broad groups of organicists must then be distinguished. The German-speaking lineage included von Ehrenfels and Köhler (*Gestalt*), von Bertalanffy, and Paul Weiss. The English form two sub groups: Haldane, Russell, Morgan, and Smuts on the one hand and Woodger, Needham, and Waddington on the other. The Americans included Ritter, Henderson, and in a less philosophical, more experimental way, E. B. Wilson and R. G. Harrison. Mention should be given to a separate development among Marxists that came through Hegel, Engels, and Marx and flowered in Soviet biology of the 1920s and early 1930s. These workers will be mentioned again in connection with Needham's intellectual affinities. Perhaps these rough divisions constitute separate paradigm groups in the Kuhnian sense. But across the national and individual differences, these men hold common views and address themselves to common problems that they felt the older perspectives dealt with poorly. All saw vitalism as part of the mechanistic paradigm rather than opposed to it because both were limited by the same images and metaphors. The

---

2. Paul Weiss claimed he was responsible for Bertalanffy's initial appreciation of the systems nature of development and behavior. Conversations took place between the two in 1927, at the same time Weiss was preparing has *Morphodynamik*. The constant concern over priority in development of modern organicism highlights the generally perceived importance of the intellectual transformations taking place in many areas of science at the same time.

organicists saw themselves as a new phenomenon working at ideas and experiments made possible only very recently by internal developments in biology and by salient intellectual transformations in other sciences, including physics and political theory. But this is not the place to reach final conclusions on the nature of paradigm groups or the adequacy of Kuhn's model in dissecting these interesting developments in biology. Rather it is time to adopt another approach, to explore the basic insights that made organicism a viable alternative approach to the organism. In the final chapter we will return to an examination of the organismic paradigm, or perhaps paradigms, in relation to mechanism and vitalism and to the perplexing dichotomy between organicism and a sophisticated neomechanism. But the remainder of this chapter will explore the elements of organicism most important to following the work of Harrison, Needham, and Weiss and to placing them in a broader intellectual context.

From an organismic perspective, the central and unavoidable focus of biology is form. Every other consideration of the biological sciences leads up to the task of at last stating the laws of organic form. Form is more than shape, more than static position of components in a whole. For biology the problem of form implies a study of genesis. How have the forms of the organic world developed? How are shapes maintained in the continual flux of metabolism? How are the boundaries of the organized events we call organisms established and maintained? Two areas of biology illustrate in an especially acute way the problem of the genesis of forms: evolution and embryology. Biological forms are grown, not assembled piecemeal. That simple fact hides the immense difficulties of accounting for the genesis of a species or of an individual. This book has focused on embryology during a period of paradigm change because here the importance of history for the content of the science itself cannot be avoided. Both stability and the emergence of novelty must be probed. The ancient debates about the nature of causality for biology and about the autonomy of biology from the physical sciences hinge on an understanding of the genesis of organic form.

In the early nineteenth century the poet Coleridge differentiated organic forms from mechanical ones according to five criteria. First, the origin of the whole precedes the differentiation of the parts. The whole is primary; the parts are derived. Second, the form manifests the process of growth by which it arose. Form and process are essentially linked, logically and historically, in organisms. Third, the organism assimilates various components into its own substance; the elements are subordinated to the whole. And fourth, the outward aspect of organisms is determined from within, by internal processes (Ritterbush 1968, pp. 20–21).

Form, according to the Romantic conception, embodies all the relations of the organism and expresses the whole and its internal organizing principles. Ritterbush argues that the Romantic conception is essentially the starting point for modern biology, not in the sense that the poets provided acceptable biological explanations or laws (which they surely did not), but in the sense that the artist and biologist face a common problem: creation of novelty and fundamental appreciation of the nature of organic form. Ritterbush points out that Goethe was among the first to use the term *morphology*, a word that has come to mean the study of shape and structure as intimately related to the processes governing form and function. Goethe remained supremely uninterested in the material substratum and processes that are obviously the soul of the matter for a biologist, but he laid out intellectually and aesthetically important parameters relevant to the science that followed him.[3]

At different critical points in the history of biology, the allegiance to concepts of organic form, borrowed heavily from poets and artists, guided the scientist's resolution of theoretical and empirical matters. I will attempt to demonstrate one such period in the first quarter of the twentieth century. Other examples alluded to have included the development of cell theory, satisfactory elucidation of the phylogenetic relations and structure of coelenterates (T. H. Huxley), and the dynamic and geometric analysis of shapes of organisms and their parts (D'Arcy Thompson). The essential relationship between biology and art should not surprise anyone. At the very beginning of biology as a systematic study, Aristotle drew heavily on the analogy of artist, artisan, and organism. The "totality of form," the composition of the elements into a functioning whole—these features gave meaning to a study of the animal. For Aristotle organic form was not limited to what we call the animate world; all of nature exhibited the characteristics of wholeness and organization. In contemporary biology, once again

3. Ritterbush 1968, p. 7. Dr. E. J. Boell, who holds the Ross G. Harrison Chair of Zoology at Yale, points out that Harrison was a devoted reader of Goethe and quoted him often.

the pit separating animate and inanimate dug in the late Renaissance with the reaction against Aristotelian science is being bridged. The construction of a virus particle is being analyzed according to architectural principles Aristotle would recognize. Formal cause, material cause, and even final cause combine to produce an understanding of the structures, particles, and intimately related functions of these elegant biological crystals.

As J. C. Kendrew points out, modern molecular biology, especially in its study of viruses, has thrown light on the intrinsic relationships of information to conformation; genetics and genesis of form are at last converging. Kendrew calls genetics the storage of information in one dimension (the sequence of bases of DNA) that is transformed into the three-dimensional structures of the organism in development. The reference to dimension, structure, and transformation shows strongly the relation of molecular studies to the essential organicism of contemporary biology (Kendrew 1968).

The connection of art and biology is forged by more than the Aristotelian analogies. Aspects of symmetry and asymmetry and construction out of fibers, spheres, and helices are also integral to the bond. Toulmin and Goodfield note that Nehemiah Grew's analysis of the structure and form of plants rested on an analogy between the organism and the fine fabric or tissue of woven fibers. Tissue metaphors have been critical to an understanding of muscle fibres and more recently of microtubules and microfilaments. Albrecht von Haller forthrightly states that "the fiber is for the physiologist what the line is for the geometer" (Toulmin and Goodfield 1962, p. 391). The globular image important for the cell theory was an alternate early analogy for the fundamental structure of matter. These strongly visualizable forms are more than props for the imagination; they have been intrinsic to explanations of basic properties of life.

Goethe felt that vision was the primary sense, the door to understanding organic form. Poetry and painting alike depended upon visual imagery and pleasing repetition of fundamental units. Goethe's interest in painting, optics, charting, and microscopic study were all aspects of his strong visual sense. Many of the visual aspects of modern science—charts, graphs, diagrams, spheres, and helices in molecular models, trees of life, fibers—owe much to Goethe's perception that "organisms could be reduced to schematic representations not just on the basis of comparisons one with another, but through the relations of their bodies of part to whole" (Ritterbush 1968, p. 6). Perception of part–whole unities was founded on a visual capacity.

Agnes Arber and C. F. A. Pantin are two contemporary writers who have again emphasized the strong relationship of art to biology rooted in the problem of form and the primacy of vision. In this context both thinkers refer to the illative sense of John Henry Newman as the corner-stone of the metaphoric consciousness in biology. The illative sense in science is related to taste in art, that is, to a sense of the appropriate. It is knowledge fused with emotion and interwoven with sense images. Both problems and resolutions, in biology as in art, arise initially in some way "from the system of images by which we represent the world in our minds" (Pantin 1968, p. 127). Arber observes that the intuition arising from the aesthetic and emotional predispositions of the scientist can be spurious and can disintegrate under the pressure of experiment, the *auto-da-fé* of all fine theories. But no true questions would exist without the intimate interplay of image, science, and art (Arber 1954). The illative sense is indispensable to biology's approach to the riddles of form because "it initiates a powerful emotional drive towards the solution of the problem, perhaps through the unconscious perception that some part or all of that system of images by which we represent the natural world to our minds, and which is the basis of our common sense, is about to undergo metamorphosis" (Pantin 1968, p. 12). Pre-cisely such a metamorphosis of image was occurring in the work of Harrison, Needham, and Weiss. Their attention to aesthetic standards and the problem of form was no accident.

Ross Harrison did not write directly about aesthetic issues, but his entire life's effort, in its content and its form, betrayed his adherence to dictates similar to the artist's. Victor Twitty, a student of Harrison at Yale, wrote of his mentor in his book *Of Scientists and Salamanders*: "If I had to identify a single factor that made Harrison's work great, I would do it in terms of esthetic considerations. He was constitutionally incapable of leaving a project until all its pieces had been fitted into a unitary whole whose composition met his artistic requirements" (1966, pp. 9–10). Harrison was dealing with questions about under-lying asymmetry in organisms, about the foundation of basic polarities, and about the course of development of organ fields.

Since the present focus is the nature of biological form, it would be instructive to see in detail how Harrison, in a 1913 paper, defined the task of anatomy. In significant respects, his world is not far from

Goethe's (Harrison 1913). Harrison begins his paper with the observation that anatomy occupies a central position among the sciences of
biology. He is concerned in his address to the American Association of
Anatomists to revive a field that had become too formal and too exclusively morphological in its methods and conception of its proper
province. In the past, anatomy had been the source of biology's finest
generalizations.

> It gave us the concept of homology or morphological equivalence
> and thereby brought order out of chaos in the matter ... of
> classifying organisms. In the cell theory, as modified by Virchow
> and Max Schultze, anatomy has made a generalization of the first
> magnitude.... By its accomplishment in the field of development
> it has related these achievements to one another, enabling us to
> formulate with precision the great problems awaiting solution.
> [pp. 403–04]

But he emphasizes that no science can live off its past. The science of
form par excellence is at a decisive turning point. The proper present
concerns of anatomy include the "field of individual development, ...
the problems of regeneration and form regulation, ... the problems of
genetics or transmission of characters, ... and lastly, the correlation
of structural mechanisms and changes therein with functional activity"
(p. 405). Biology seeks to understand the interdependencies of phenomena.

Far from seeing anatomy as a static science, Harrison stated the
nature of this morphological science as follows:

> Anatomy must, in short, busy itself with all phases of the problem
> of organic form. It will be found that they are as fundamental as,
> and perhaps even more recondite than, are the problems of func-
> tion. Recent opinion on the origin of life serves but to show how
> supposedly fundamental distinctions, as to function, between
> living and non-living matter fade when subjected to close scrutiny,
> and it may well turn out that the morphological quality of specific
> form with heterogeneity of material, arising gradually from a
> relatively specific germ, is after all the most peculiar property of
> living matter.... Organic form is the product of protoplasmic
> activity and must, therefore, find its explanation in the dynamics
> of living matter, but *it is the mystery and beauty of organic form that sets*

the problem for us. Structure is a product of function, and yet at the same time, is the basis of function. The activities of an organism may be nothing more than continuance of those changes that produce development. [pp. 405–06, italics added]

Harrison defines form as the totality of relationships of a developing organism. An approach to nature aided by a combination of the illative sense and analytic rationality is evident in Harrison's statement. He insists that organic form cannot be static, fixed. "A statical organism can only be a dead organism . . . , and dead organisms mean dead science" (p. 406).

Nor can the science that investigates form rely on ideal, comparative schemes. Harrison spends the last part of his paper trying to obliterate the gulf in methodology between physiology and anatomy. The essence of his organicism is a new appreciation of interconnectedness of structure and function in developing animals. He pleads for an experimental approach to the problem of form, for a concretization of its principles. In his emphasis on experiment and analysis Harrison is in a different world from Goethe. The embryologist is essentially interested in the precise materials and processes of development, not simply in the aesthetic perceptions that give his efforts meaning and motive. "Organic form must find its explanation in the dynamics of matter, and the distinction between living and non-living must fade." Aristotle would approve of Harrison; both know that the most peculiar quality of life is that "morphological quality of specific form with heterogeneity of material." The structure–function and part–whole relations, understood in a constant dialectic interplay, constitute the cornerstone of the developmental edifice.

Joseph Needham contributed a paper to Lancelot Law Whyte's *Aspects of Form* that sums up his long-held beliefs about the nature of organic form and the methods adopted by biology to explore it (Needham 1951, pp. 77–91). He begins with a tribute to D'Arcy Thompson and a discussion of the role of mathematics in the science of form, a constant thread in Needham's writing. If Aristotle is most congenial to Harrison, Plato dominates the soul of Needham.[4] The double debt

---

4. Needham is a complex fabric of Aristotelian and Platonic fibers. He notes that biochemistry has more affinities with Aristotle because of an intense consciousness of matter, which always had at least a minimum of form in its constitution from the four elements. And for the modern chemist, form permeates the whole of the science.

is significant for the nature of the organic mechanism or nonvitalist
organicism that both men were building. Yet Needham felt there was
something missing from D'Arcy Thompson's exclusively mathematical
treatment, something that left the mansion of biology, swept clean by
mathematics, open still to possession by demons of vitalism.

> While no one could possibly underestimate the magnitude of the
> task performed by D'Arcy Thompson, it was nevertheless, in spite
> of all its mathematical profundity, less difficult in a way than the
> problem of finding some relation between the gross morphological
> forms manifested by living things and the specific molecular con-
> stitutions which they possess.

The effort to bridge "this terrifying intellectual gap" was the soul of
his own approach to form (Needham 1951, p. 78).

Whitehead is an important philosopher for Needham's conception
of his task. His organic materialism emphasized the primacy of organism over atom. Therefore, "the old controversies about the reduci-
bility or irreducibility of biological facts to physical-chemical facts are
now seen to be unnecessary if we realize that we have to deal with
different levels of organization. The task of science is to elucidate the
regularities which occur at each of these levels..." (p. 78). Connection
between levels and development from one level of complexity to the
next are the key foci of organicist biology. Again, form is conceived as
the totality of structured relationships unfolded in development. Central to this conception are the dual categories of organization and
energy, which are Needham's modern equivalents of Aristotelian form
and matter.

It remained impossible to connect biochemistry with morphology as
long as concepts of structure were poorly developed in chemistry itself.
Naïve reductionism remained a possibility if there were still some
simple, unorganized entity in terms of which "higher structure" could
be explained. Needham remarks that it was possible until World War I
to be skeptical about the reality of structure on the chemical level. He
cites the pioneering importance of Langmuir's and Harkin's experiments on monomolecular films. Spatial relations of realistically conceived molecules became critical to an understanding of the properties
of biological membranes. Analysis of biological molecules by X-ray
crystallography added immeasurably to the appreciation of structure
at the finest dimensions of the organism. This work dates from the 1920s

study of polysaccharides by Sponsler in California. Soon after, Astbury and his school at Leeds began research on animal textile fibers, work that led rather directly to modern structural analysis of many important proteins.

In an article entitled "Fifty years of progress in structural chemistry and molecular biology," Linus Pauling, a central figure in several basic advances in the understanding of molecular structure in this century, illuminates the extent and nature of the difficulties to be resolved before the idea of form at the most "fundamental" level was clear (1970). Without the progress in understanding molecular organization outlined by Pauling, the new biological conception of structure–function relationships would have remained radically incomplete. Pauling calls the 100 years from 1780 to 1880 the period of development for the classical theory of chemical structure. In the decades after 1880 those ideas were clarified and the principles of thermodynamics and statistical mechanics were applied to chemical problems. But in 1920 the nature of the chemical bond was largely a mystery. In 1926, a year after the first appearance of the theory of quantum mechanics, Pauling began to apply the powerful new theory to the study of the structure of molecules. Near the end of the 1920s covalent and ionic bonds were understood in the sense that the properties of molecules were explicable in terms of structure. Furthermore, structure itself came to be seen as a problem of systems, and so of function, on all levels.

Pauling dates his direct interest in biological molecules from 1935. The structure of proteins was solved in the following years in favor of the polypeptide chain theory.[5] A few years later Pauling proposed the fruitful model of the alpha helix in proteins, thus clarifying the idea of repeating subunits as the basis of complex structure. Pauling nearly proposed the correct structure for DNA and was certainly responsible for laying out the principles applied so well by Watson and Crick (Pauling and Delbrück 1940). These concepts were crucial for non-reductionist molecular biology, in which the paradox of field and particle could be approached.

While biophysics continued to penetrate molecular structure, many

5. Dorothy Wrinch, an important member of the Theoretical Biology Club, had supported the ring theory of protein structure. Her role in Needham's appreciation of molecular structure will be discussed more thoroughly in a later chapter.

of its fruits were applied from the beginning. Needham considered the study of muscle fibers fundamental to forging the link between form and metabolism. An architectural component of the muscle fiber itself, myosin, was found to change shape during contraction. Myosin was seen at the same time as a contractile protein and as the enzyme that liberated the energy necessary for contraction from ATP. Needham concluded that "it would seem that this state of affairs in muscle has extremely important implications for morphology in general and morphogenesis in particular"(1941, p. 82). Physical structure was altered by function and vice versa. However, Joseph Needham worked not on muscle, but on another aspect of the synthesis of chemistry and morphogenesis.[6] He focused his attention in the 1930s on "morphogenetic hormones," which he hoped would reveal the nature of induction phenomena discovered in Hans Spemann's laboratory in Germany. Induction is surely much more complicated than Needham felt in those years, but his theoretical point rests unperturbed: "The foundations of morphological form are to be sought in the proteins responsible for cell-structure, and ... these are inescapably connected with the normal metabolic processes of the living cell as a going concern" (1951, p. 86).

Harrison's appreciation of the primacy of form was exemplified by his attitude to anatomy as a science, and Needham clarified his own position in a paper directed to biochemical aspects of form and growth. Paul Weiss took a more direct approach and explicitly discussed the relation of form in biology and art in the article "Beauty and the beast" (1955). The rule of order over randomness was the foundation of the sense of beauty. The rule was expressed by features such as symmetry, repetition, and alteration of elements. Patterns were of both space and time, of both structure and process. Weiss compared the patterns perceived as beautiful in human artifacts and in organisms and concluded that the perceptions were based on a common viewpoint: "In the last analysis, whatever organic form we view has had a history and has come to be what it is through sequences of developmental processes" (p. 287). In concert with Goethe and Coleridge, Weiss ascribed the properties of organic form to both the products of human creation and the works of nature. They further agreed that

6. His wife, Dorothy Needham, was an active researcher in muscle biochemistry at Cambridge. Her book (1972) on the history of the biochemistry of muscle contraction is indispensable.

the central issue was the primacy of ordered internal growth over piecemeal assembly of machine forms. Weiss noted that what we perceive as static and final is a product "of measured orderliness of the developmental actions and interactions by which it has come about. . . . Goethe called architecture 'frozen music.' In the same sense, organic form is frozen development; and formal beauty reflects developmental order" (p. 288). He went on to discuss growth of tree rings, shells, and skeletal components. Various geometrical forms repeat themselves in the organic world. The same forms appear on Japanese scrolls, Gothic ironwork, and many works of architecture. Systems of lines or points, arranged in geometrically regular arrays, betray their rules of genesis. It is hardly surprising that Weiss found his life's work in unraveling rules of order in developmental biology.

Weiss believed that physical models illuminated the patterns presented by organisms. He would have been at home with Bütschli's foam models of protoplasm, and he cited with approval the work of Runge on chemical reactions resulting in patterns on filter paper. Again we are reminded of the basic aesthetic units of fibers, spheres, helices, and the tissues woven from them. Orderly dynamics yields aesthetic design. Near the conclusion of his paper, Weiss stressed the notion of emergent order, but its mystery is dissipated in favor of a concrete formulation.

> These same principles, however, reappear in larger dimensions as the self-ordering of systems of particles in cells, or cells in tissues, or parts in organisms, or even organisms in a group. Wherever we study such emergent order, we recognize it to be of tripartite origin, involving (i) elements with inner order, (ii) their orderly interactions, and (iii) an environment fit to sustain their ordered group behavior. [p. 288]

The world of Coleridge has come to fruition in a biological organicism.

Problems of form grade naturally into a consideration of symmetry, polarity, and pattern. An understanding of these three elements is critical to an appreciation of nonmechanist paradigms throughout the history of biology. The significance of each component was transformed radically in the articulation of modern organicism. Harrison, Needham, and Weiss each believed that symmetry relations of organisms rested on a fundamental asymmetry at the molecular core. Asymmetry in organisms has historically been a cornerstone for theories of vitalism. Inorganic nature was widely felt to be the province of regular symmetry relations; the organic world was conceived as the realm of extraordinary spatial forms, such as the logarithmic spiral of *Nautilus* shells and the fivefold radial symmetry of starfish. Neither shape can be reduced to the simple geometry of crystalline space lattices. Crystals manifesting simple geometrical shapes surely were products of the laws of chemistry and physics, but the peculiar symmetries and asymmetries of organisms seemed to call for unique organizing principles.

Not only the molecules found in organisms but their spatial relationships and the connection of both substance and form to function and growth, were at issue in decisions about paradigms.[7] In 1826 Wöhler, along with Liebig, observed that cyanic and fulminic acid have the same percentage composition. This work laid the foundation for development of the principle of isomerism, an indispensable step in the process of applying concepts of form to the chemical level. Studying isomerism is tantamount to studying transformations of form. But instead of undermining vitalistic doctrines, investigation of isomerism led for a time to a complex support for theories of unique, nonmaterial directive agencies in living nature. This support came ironically from the work of Louis Pasteur, remembered for his successful attack on doctrines of spontaneous generation. Pasteur himself did not come to fully vitalistic positions in relation to his studies on stereo-isomerism, but he delineated the key terms of the controversy.

During the years 1844–49 Pasteur worked on the optical isomers of tartaric acid. Chemists knew that certain quartz crystals could be divided into two groups whose members are related to each other as object is to image. Herschel had suggested in 1820 that the difference in optical activity of the quartz crystals might be related to their opposite symmetries.[8] Pasteur noted that crystals of the tartarates possessed

7. A similar mistake is made in modern biochemistry and genetics when it is assumed that knowledge of the genetic code automatically generates understanding of pattern and form if one were only clever enough. The full organicist perspective of molecular biology, including molecular genetics, is necessary to approach the form and genesis dimensions. A good example of an organismic study on this level is the work of Racker on genetics, assembly, and function of subcellular organelles (see Bruni and Racker 1968). The *Journal for Biological Chemistry* for 1969, volume 244, continues a series of articles by Racker and his associates on reconstitution of the mitochondrial electron transport system and resolution of functional structures of chloroplasts.

8. Optical activity refers to the property of certain substances, for example, a crystal of iceland spar, of polarizing a beam of light passed through the substance. Biot had observed in 1815 that solutions as well as crystals were capable of rotating the plane of polarization of light. The search for the structural basis of optical activity was the context in which Pasteur undertook his work on tartaric acid (see McPhearson 1917).

opposite planes of symmetry, similar to those of quartz. Solutions of tartarate made up from one type of crystal rotated the plane of light to the right (dextrorotatory), while solutions made up from crystals of opposite symmetry rotated light to the left (levorotatory). Relating the effects of dextro- and levotartaric acid[9] to the asymmetrical character of their molecules was a fundamental step in understanding the role of asymmetries in nature.

An asymmetric compound prepared in the laboratory is obtained in the inactive form, that is, as a *mixture* of the two optically active forms. But in organic nature an asymmetric compound almost always exists in the active form. Pasteur remarked in a speech before the Chemical Society of Paris in 1860 that this difference is the most critical distinction between "living" and "dead" nature (McPhearson 1917, p. 77). Organisms have the power to take inactive materials such as carbon dioxide and water and to produce preferentially one optically active substance to the exclusion of all other possible forms. The problem of why mixtures are not found in nature is analogous to Driesch's. Driesch was puzzled by the capacity of his "harmonious equipotential system," the seemingly homogeneous egg or isolated early blastomere, to grow into the complex patterns of the adult. The essential issue for Driesch became the observed power of regulation in organisms. On the chemical level the problem was how to account for specific asymmetry from an indifferent starting point.

F. R. Japp, in an address to the British Association in 1898 on "Stereochemistry and vitalism," drew vividly the vitalistic conclusion: only a directive, nonmaterial, intelligent force would be capable of selecting the particular molecular dissymmetries found in organic nature (1898). Japp's lecture started a controversy in which the issues were gradually clarified. Regulation of form, on the chemical as well as on the whole embryo level, was again the stumbling block. By 1912 several partially asymmetric syntheses had been achieved in the laboratory. However, the importance of such refutations of the vitalist assertions was weakened by the fact that in each case some molecule originally derived from an organism, either an enzyme or another optically active compound, was used in the synthesis. Since it became clear that living systems could maintain their peculiar specific processes

9. Here the prefixes *dextro-* and *levo-* refer to the spatial forms of the crystals, not to the direction of rotation of the plane of polarized light. It is not necessarily true that crystals of left-hand symmetry rotate light to the left.

given the proper starting conditions, the problem reduced to how the *first* asymmetrical natural synthesis occurred. That is, in organic nature since the origin of life, "the 'asymmetric forces' of Pasteur need *not* be looked for *outside* the organism, for they are determined by the chemical system *in* its cells" (Jaeger 1917, p. 288). Even the question of the origin of specific asymmetries lost its baffling quality in principle because several possible schemes for the generation of optically active compounds in preliving nature were advanced, ranging from the operation of an asymmetrical physical force such as gravity to the chance concentration of several molecules of the same symmetry determining the further reactions possible in a semiclosed system. In 1894, even before Japp's lecture, E. Fischer had pointed out that syntheses outside living cells were not totally random in relation to symmetry properties. He felt Pasteur's original distinction between "living" and "dead" was too extreme. Laboratory syntheses do not yield all possible stereoisomers but only a few; thus these reactions show some preferential quality (McPhearson 1917).

The final appreciation of asymmetric synthesis awaits full understanding on a molecular level of the origin of life. The purpose of the above discussion was not to settle the ultimate issues of organic form but to point out the intricate nature of the problem. The discussion of symmetry could have focused on several questions instead of on the controversy over stereochemistry and vitalism. But the debate was typical and fundamental to the understanding of form in Harrison's approach to the postulated molecular asymmetry in the limb field, to Needham's hypothesis of anisomorphic micelles relevant to gastrulation, and to Weiss's understanding of tissue fabrics. The link among the three men was their use of the idea of liquid crystals, which was conditioned by the approach taken to molecular asymmetry. It was evident by the early twentieth century that outside directive forces need not be invoked. Rather than rehashing the old arguments for mechanism or vitalism, the issue of symmetry on a molecular level was better approached from an organicist perspective. Just as the problem of form (development of complex asymmetry from simpler starting situations) was analogous for the embryologist and the biochemist, so too fruitful answers transcended the former categories of organic and inorganic. Harrison, Needham, and Weiss each worked out for himself a view of symmetry on a fine structure level that was critical to his theoretical and experimental perspectives.

It is a short step from a consideration of symmetry to that of polarity. Here, however, the focus will be on the level of calls and embryos. Lewis Wolpert, a contemporary British biologist, has recently re-emphasized studies of polarity in a way which clarifies the organismic paradigm (1970, pp. 198–230).

Wolpert defines polarity as an ordering relationship that involves a system of coordinates with directional information. Polarity specifies direction of measurement. He reexamines the older work on hydroids and sea urchin embryos in order to show the rich possibilities for analysis of "positional information" and "polarity potential" (p. 225). Relating these properties to older ideas of fields, Wolpert attempts to concretize the concepts in intriguing ways. For example, he speculates that fields[10] probably are never larger than fifty cells long and that time courses for specifying positional information can be closely determined with modern biochemical techniques and could be related to gene functioning. Wolpert highlights the importance of the old theme of polarity by showing how it can be approached conceptually and experimentally today. As he points out, little work has been done since the 1920s and 1930s that has changed biology's grasp of the issues. By that time, postulated mechanisms of pattern formation had been related, or the attempt had been made to relate them, to ideas of polarity, gradient, and field. The precise nature of these concepts will be sketched in the discussions on the approach Harrison, Needham, and Weiss made to pattern problems. Here it is useful to outline the history of the idea of polarity in developmental biology from about 1900 to 1940.

Theodor Boveri's (1862–1915) fundamental goal was to determine the physiological relationships between all structure and cell processes. Appropriately, he was among the first biologists to call attention to the importance of gradients and polarity in animal development.[11] In

10. Wolpert defines a field as a system with all its positional information specified with respect to the same point or points of reference. Wolpert's paper translates the language of the older work on pattern and polarity into systems terminology. The translation is not a trivial restatement; instead it shows that the basic premises of a biological structuralism can be found in the work of a generation ago. Wolpert draws heavily from Child, Hörstaduis, and Dalcq. He concentrates on the fundamental nature of gradients and polarity in biology at a time when many workers have lost track of the form problem in the flush of triumph in molecular genetics interpreted from a neomechanist perspective.

11. Gradient and polarity are not synonomous, but the ideas are usually closely related. Polarity here refers to the directional properties of a gradient, whether the gradient be of substances or processes.

his 1901 studies on sea urchin eggs, Boveri noted that the isolated upper portion was not capable of gastrulating, but the lower or vegetal portion could gastrulate (Oppenheimer 1967, pp. 78–86). He developed the idea of a privileged region of dominance as a causal factor in development. Hans Spemann acknowledged a debt to Boveri's work on stratification in eggs for his own ideas about gradients and polarity (Spemann 1938, pp. 142, 341). Boveri introduced the term *Gefälle*, or gradient, into modern biology. Spemann calls Boveri's conception the "general gradient theory" to differentiate it from the narrower theory of Child. The essence of Boveri's theory was that "the body of many, if not all animals, at least in the embryonic state, possesses one or several axes with unequal poles along which there exists a gradient of some sort. The course of development depends on these gradients to a high degree."[12]

Gradients came into full prominence with the work of C. M. Child. His concept of activity gradients based on metabolic rate and underlying other phenomena of morphogenesis was popularized, particularly in England, by Huxley and DeBeer in their widely read text of 1934.[13] They generalized Child's gradients into the idea of "gradient fields." Child believed there was, as a quite general phenomenon in development, a primary center of activity determining a quantitative metabolic gradient. New centers of activity could arise as a result of physiological isolation. The focal idea was that morphological structures derived from physiological *processes* (Spemann 1938, p. 325; Child 1941, esp. chap. 8). With his emphasis on activity and process, Child opposed the idea that intimate protoplasmic structure was the primary determinate of pattern. Rather, such things as crystalline structures derived from

12. Spemann 1938, p. 318 (see also Boveri 1901). It is especially appropriate to cite Boveri in connection with polarity aspects of biology's form problem. Many of Boveri's beautiful and fruitful interpretations of the role of chromosomes in heredity were based on an appreciation of form and organized structure. Boveri felt that the *picture* or image was essential to biology, and not simply a means of representation. He himself was a master draftsman and painted with considerable proficiency. His emphasis on the picture was a counterinfluence to a simplistic mechanistic assumption that chemistry would solve all biology's puzzles. Boveri appreciated that form was no more alien to chemistry than to biology and that nonvitalist explanations had to deal with organized structures wherever they appeared. Boveri is a good example of the working of the visual and illative senses in science. For a discussion of his life, art, and biology, see Baltzer 1967.

13. Child originally based his theoretical interpretations on work on hydroids and planaria. Huxley and DeBeer generalized it to apply to Spemann's system and to the amphibian egg as a whole. Child seems to have accepted the wider applications of his interpreters.

metabolism. He felt that "there is, at present, no evidence for, and much against, the concept of organismic pattern as primarily a pattern of molecular structure and orientation" (1941, p. 699). Instead, the asymmetries of organisms were related to more general earlier patterns. Child criticized the analogy of crystal and organism for "putting the cart before the horse." He summed up his own position as follows: "The effective factor in development appears beyond question to be metabolism; concentration gradients, molecular arrangements, and morphological pattern are apparently results of earlier metabolic patterns, though all of them, when present, may become factors in modifying these patterns" (p. 705).

Child's critique of the crystal analogy in biology was significant. He thought that the gradient system alone was sufficient to provide the organizing principles of a developing system. Believing the "whole is more than the sum of its parts," Child was not a traditional mechanist. The wholeness consisted of the gradient pattern and the relations of dominance and subordination arising from it (p. 703). Child did not integrate his hypothesis of process underlying spatial and temporal pattern with an appreciation of the intimate structure of the cell and organism. A key to his failure is rejection of the crystal analogy in its nonmechanist sense of intermediate level of organization in which structure and function come together without argument over priorities. The following treatment of Harrison should make plain how his conception differed from Child's. Harrison took a profitable approach to biological gradients and polarity that still underlies good contemporary work. The common criticism of gradient concepts that pervades discussion in current developmental biology is relevant to Child's framework, but not to Harrison's.

Considerations of symmetry, polarity, and gradient are part of a general treatment of pattern. The single most important organizing principle developed in this century to treat pattern was that of *field*. It is impossible to delay any longer a preliminary consideration of how field ideas have functioned in biology. Alexander Gurwitsch in 1922 was the first writer to use the term in biology (1922).[14] A few years later

14. Victor Hamburger suggested to Jane Oppenheimer in conversation that Ross Harrison was probably the first to introduce explicitly the concept of fields into embryology. But Harrison was always careful of terminology, anxious to make sure a new word carried definite meaning, and he surely did not elaborate the major axes of field theory. His study of the newt limb is a classic instance of analysis of the structure of a field, probably still the most careful and provocative work on the subject. But the most dramatic field biology before Gurwitsch was developed in the last chapter of D'Arcy Thompson's 1917 *On Growth and Form*.

Paul Weiss used field concepts to explain the results of his and others' work on limb regeneration in amphibians (1926). Weiss, having been trained as an engineer, brought into biology the early thinking on systems. Well grounded in the physical sciences, he brought to biology intellectual frameworks derived from the late nineteenth and early twentieth century study of electromagnetic fields and light-wave propogation. In addition to physics, another major source of field ideas for developmental biology was psychology, especially the work of von Ehrenfels and Wolfgang Köhler. Gestalt psychology, developed in opposition to the classic associationist theories of perception, stressed wholes and regulation, the two perennial stumbling blocks for embryological investigation. A third source of field concepts is biology itself, in particular the work of Harrison on symmetry and laterality in the developing limb and the speculation on gradients outlined above.

It is important to glance at the physical context in which field thinking took root. Whitehead notes that field and particle are classic antithetical notions in Western science and philosophy. They are not logically contradictory, but normally explanation in terms of atoms has excluded explanation in terms of "action at a distance" or continua. However, by the end of the nineteenth century both sorts of ideas were indispensable. Ordinary matter was thought of as atomic; electromagnetic phenomena were conceived as arising from a continuous field (Whitehead 1925, p. 94). Two sorts of fields were indispensable to physics by the date of Gurwitsch's paper in 1922: gravitational and electromagnetic. Later atomic physics would require field concepts for weak and strong interactions between subatomic particles. As Einstein and Infeld make clear in their popular exposition, *The Evolution of Physics*, fields had a clear operational meaning based on the behavior of objects placed within otherwise "empty space" (1938). The radical sense of true action at a distance across empty space was never intended by the biological fields of Harrison, Needham, or Weiss. Undoubtedly biological field thought was rooted in physical theories, but the purely physical notion, requiring empty space, if pushed to its logical consequences would lead to an essentially vitalist position. For Harrison, Needham, and Weiss, the position effects requiring concepts of wholeness and regulation were always linked to biochemistry. The same was definitely not true for Driesch, but he did not develop his theory in a field context. Gurwitsch is less clear about the material status of his fields.

Historically the crystal analogy abides in atomic conceptions.

Opposition to the analogy in an explanatory role came from organicist thinking. Field notions as developed in biology were meant to bridge the gap between the polar opposites. To do so necessitated rethinking several historical dichotomies such as structure and function, crystal and organism, part and whole. The organicist biology developed by Harrison, Needham, and Weiss found a way beyond the antithesis; organism and organization required a union of field and particle.

Wolfgang Köhler, the founder of Gestalt psychology, was inspired by the field phenomena of physics and saw in them a way beyond the additive framework of classic psychology prevailing from Locke into the contemporary period (1947). A crucial concept for Gestalt psychology is that of *configuration*. Von Ehrenfels had defined configurations as psychical states whose properties cannot be obtained by placing together the characteristics of the parts. He developed criteria according to which configurations could be transposed. The analogy implied is to a musical theme that can be put into different keys without losing its essential features. Köhler noted that typical configurations occurred in physical systems, in particular the distribution of a charge on an electric conductor. He hoped to show that psychical states were special cases of physical configurations (Bertalanffy 1933, p. 51). In the late 1920s Köhler applied Gestalt theory to embryological problems. He emphasized that the whole whose primacy over its parts changed their character, could not be understood by an additive process. Köhler did not consider biology an autonomous science. In fact his goal was the opposite, that is, to show that psychology was a special case of physics.[15]

Köhler saw Gestalt theory as a third way beyond the limitations of mosaic mechanist theories and the supraorganismic principles of vitalism. Driesch's contention that position effects are observable only in living organisms was wrong; that properties and functions of parts

---

15. Paul Weiss corresponded with Köhler in the 1920s on the basis of their common interest in field phenomena. In a conversation on August 1, 1970, Dr. Weiss said he met Köhler at the 1927 International Congress of Genetics. Weiss's publication of *Morphodynamik* had preceded the congress by a year. He noted that many biologists were thinking in field-like terms independently of direct analogy with physics or psychology. Any phenomenon not comprehended by mosaic explanations is a good candidate for field concepts. Weiss said he and Köhler independently came to the notion of fields from physics, but they later diverged in their use of the concepts. Köhler pushed further his analogies with such systems as conductors whereas Weiss thought more and more in biological terms, finding the suggestiveness of electric phenomena limited in embryology, partly because of the paradoxically vitalist implications.

depend on position within the whole is a fundamental property of many structures. The key concept for Köhler was equilibrium. Every system to which the second law of thermodynamics applies sooner or later reaches equilibrium. An organism can be considered a physical configuration with properties of wholeness that depend upon the inner dynamical properties of the system, that is, upon the fact that the momentary state of every part determines that of the other parts. Self-regulation of organisms follows from principles of Gestalt because in a system with several degrees of freedom, the occurrences in every partial region are under the control of the whole (Bertalanffy 1933, pp. 102–08). Köhler sought in inorganic systems the principles that would explain regulation in organisms. Regulation concerns direction and goals, that is, the solution to regulation involves a solution to teleology. Only if the initial conditions of a system are altered too severely will the system fail to achieve its "goal." Different initial conditions would yield different processes, regulations, and final states. But in any case, control of the system parts by the state of the whole is inevitable.

Objections to Gestalt theory in embryology centered around the absence of fixed structural conditions in developing biological forms. An electrical conductor was an inappropriate analogy because its shape was fixed and the system as a whole did not have a history. A biological organicism would have to deal head on with novelty as well as wholeness. Thus, introduction of concepts of hierarchy, levels, and constrained pathways of development basically separated men such as Weiss and Needham from Köhler.

About 1941 Gurwitsch began to explore an organic formative factor that he called *Morphe*. By the early 1920s he abandoned this concept for that of fields and focused on form regulation in the flower head of the camomille and the mushroom. The field concept was useful because there was no evident differentiation of the structural units of the fungus, yet resultant shapes were highly regular and specific. Gurwitsch's fields stressed geometrical properties and constituted stimulus fields rather than fields of force. The source and extent of the field were not confined to the material of the organism in question. Its center could well be some geometric point outside the plant. In his effort to go beyond pure chemical theories and theories based on cellular determination, Gurwitsch successfully avoided a vitalistic explanation of the difficult forms of the mushroom in which an originally irregular growing material takes on a simple geometrical form. He was interested in showing that there were physical realities corresponding to the terms in his analytical formulas, but chemical theories were logically and practically excluded. A field was a way of connecting vectors that controlled spatial transformations. Gurwitsch was initially occupied only with surfaces of organisms, that is, with external shapes and contours. The purpose was to explain form without relying on mutual interaction of parts. In that way a great variety of forms constructed from essentially similar parts (e.g., different bones) or very similar forms from various parts could be understood (Bertalanffy 1933, pp. 112–18).

The strong geometrical orientation dematerialized Gurwitsch's fields much more than Harrison, Needham, or Weiss would permit. Gurwitsch's fields lacked grounding in biochemistry less from an analogy to radical physical concepts than from his Platonic trust in geometry. His solution to the form problem was mathematical, not physical or biological.[16]

Paul Weiss objected to the ideal fields of Gurwitsch, which were based not on the immense structural complexity of the organism but on ideal geometric constructions. Weiss's field concept will be examined in detail later. Here it is important to note that his organicism required paying strict attention to intimate structure and chemistry (and thus particle explanations) as well as to continua, lines of force, and position effects (and thus field explanations). Weiss conceived of a field as a system of organizing factors that proceed from already organized parts to other regions and that result in formation of typical patterns. Fields break up during development, producing a number of subfields that direct development of organs within the organism. He attempted to draw up field laws describing such processes. In sum, a field was the complex of "factors which *cause the originally indefinite course of the individual parts of a germ to become definite and specific*, and, furthermore, cause this to occur *in compliance with a typical pattern*" (Weiss 1939, p. 290 [italics in orig.]) The status of his field laws was in constant question. Weiss attempted to eliminate confusion by emphasizing that the field concept was "an abstraction trying to give expression to a group of phenomena observed in living systems." It was descriptive, not analytical and causal. Its roots were empirical, and the task facing

16. For a later discussion of his fields, see Gurwitsch 1927.

the embryologist was to concretize the concept, to link the symbolic terms with the physical germ. The field concept was meant to stimulate further research, not to provide a verbal explanation where full understanding was lacking.[17]

C. H. Waddington has made an effort to clarify the field concept further and to show its current usefulness. During the 1930s Waddington introduced the idea of the individuation field to describe a field associated with the formation of a definite organ with characteristic individual shape. He cautioned against using the term to refer to a region or district without meaning to designate the "co-ordinated and integrated character of the whole complex of processes" (1956, p. 25). Definite spatial relation of processes was the key notion. Waddington drew the analogy between his individuation field and the behavior of magnetic or other physical fields.

> For instance, if a field is cut in two each half may reconstitute a complete field, so that two whole organs are developed. These are often mirror images of one another. On the other hand, if two fields are brought together and allowed to fuse, they may rearrange themselves into a single field. Again, if a part of a field, either central or peripheral, is removed, the remainder may compensate for the defect and become complete again, while the isolated part can often become modified into a small but complete field.[18]

However, Waddington was not content with physical analogies and

17. Weiss 1939, p. 292. It is worthwhile stressing Weiss's warning that field concepts were largely descriptive; their value remained to be proved in a causal sense. The value of his organicism, in contrast to the alternative mechanism–vitalism paradigm, was precisely in the effort to concretize, to avoid verbal excuse, and to unify previously disparate concepts and experiments. The field work of the 1930s is much maligned for having inhibited progress in embryology. The question is confused, but viewing the work from the perspective of building an organismic biology to bridge old dichotomies removes much of the legitimacy of the criticism.

18. 1956, pp. 27–28 (see also Waddington 1934). Waddington worked with Needham throughout the 1930s, and their thought on field problems was closely correlated. It is interesting to notice that Waddington as well as Weiss came to biology from other areas: Waddington from geology, Weiss from engineering. That Waddington has progressively come to see the idea of field as an essentially topographical notion and that Weiss went from fields to fully mature systems thinking are comprehensible developments. Needham also came to the embryological world from another discipline, that is, from biochemistry. His contribution to the growing new organicist paradigm lay in an attempted unification of chemistry and form. Most valuable statements of field concepts came from such amphibious thinkers. The nature of the problems of embryology made convergence of disciplines inevitable.

has continued to argue that field theory has a specific meaning in biology. There is only one type of gravitational field and one sort of electromagnetic field, but there are almost as many potential biological fields as there are organs and species. What is necessary if the concept of field is to be useful at all, even in a descriptive sense, is an understanding of how fields are transposed and modified to produce the observed heterogeneity. This task is a variation of that undertaken by D'Arcy Thompson. Waddington's effort to make the concept of field precise has led him into the realm of topology, where he has been guided by René Thom (1970).[19]

Waddington states that the idea of field requires reference to a multidimensional space, "which would have axes on which one could plot not only position in time and the three dimensions of space but also concentrations of essential chemical compounds" (1966, p. 109). His basic concept is that of a chreod, a directed path, or a trajectory of normal development. The concept is introduced to deal with the causal complexity of fields and to stress their regulative character. Displaced points are brought back into place by the "attractor surface" of the chreod. If a point escapes the attractor surface, a new situation exists in which regulation is disturbed and a different final state is to be expected. The strength of the canalization of a developmental chreod can be tested by experimental means: breeding and genetics, transplantation, fusion of parts, and defect experiments. Canalization refers to degree of regulation. The idea of a chreod is tremendously suggestive but hardly a simplification of the problem. Realization of the number of relevant vector fields or dimensions that have to be considered in characterizing an embryo dispels hope for immediate solution of specific problems. Waddington stresses the importance, but also the limitations, of his excursion into theoretical biology. An embryological field is more complex than electromagnetic or gravitational fields in two ways: time can never be left out of the picture and the material substratum is immensely more complicated. Use of the chreod concept is only appropriate when regulation is an issue.

19. The Theoretical Biology Club of the 1930s, which included Needham and Waddington, emphasized that the form problem of biology would have to use the insights of topology and looked to the thought of D'Arcy Thompson as a first step in that direction. The early hopes have been largely unfulfilled, partly because of the difficulty of the task, partly from lack of theoretical vision. Thom stresses that his models say nothing of a causal nature but only indicate the possibility of a description of developing organic forms with topological methods.

Any such regulative properties can be expressed by specifying some "normal" developmental pathway within a multidimensional space and describing the manner in which it acts as an attractor for neighboring pathways. A region of phase space characterized by an attractor time trajectory has been called a chreod. A developmental field is essentially a chreod, whereas electromagnetic and stationary gravitational fields are not. [p. 123]

Thus the notion of field has been developed from Köhler's first simple analogy to Waddington's highly sophisticated one. Proper use of fields in biology requires understanding of organization, increasing complexity, hierarchy, and transformations over time. It is precisely these characteristics that lead to the suggestion that organicist biology, growing out of work by Harrison, Needham, Waddington, Weiss, and others, is a type of structuralism related to similar frameworks in many areas. Organicist structuralism is a third way to deal with form, organization, and regulation; it is different from both the additive point of view (mechanism) and from philosophies of emergence (vitalism). The paradigm switch in embryology taking shape in the first half of this century consisted of the adoption of a structuralist perspective. The best way to support this contention is to focus on form and field problems.

Jean Piaget, the Swiss psychologist, has defined structuralism and attempted to indicate the similarities among structuralist approaches in different disciplines (1971; see also 1967a). A structure "is a system of transformations. Inasmuch as it is a system and not a mere collection of elements and their properties, these transformations involve laws: the structure is preserved or enriched by the interplay of its transformation laws. . . . In short, the notion of structure is comprised of three key ideas: the idea of *wholeness*, the idea of *transformation*, and the idea of *self-regulation*" (1971, p. 5 [italic added]).

The question of form is central to structuralism. Shape is approached not from a sense of static anatomy but from an appreciation of systematic and dynamic transformation and conservation of the totality. A whole is present if the elements of a structure are subordinated to the laws characterizing the system as such. Such laws cannot be reducible to cumulative associations but "confer on the whole as such over-all properties distinct from the properties of its elements" (p. 7). Piaget withholds the designation of *structure* (whole) from the Gestalt configuration because the latter gave insufficient rigorous attention to the origin of laws of composition and to transformations, that is, Gestalt theory neglected history. Weiss diverged from Köhler precisely on the matter of history. Gestalt fields were static forms because they relied too heavily on physical analogies. Biological fields required serious attention to genesis. For Piaget's structuralism, the important issue is neither the element nor some whole imposed upon the parts, but the relations among elements. The processes of composition demand exact attention; the whole is nothing more than the resultant of these relations or compositions, whose laws are those of the system. Whitehead's event is a structuralist conception, and the biological organism is a structure par excellence.

There is a bipolarity at the heart of the notion of structure. If the defining aspect of structured wholes lies in laws of composition,

> these laws must of their very nature be *structuring*; it is the constant duality, or bipolarity, of always being simultaneously *structuring* and *structured* that accounts for the success of the notion of law or rule. ... Like Cournot's "order" (a special case of the structures treated in modern algebra), a structure's laws of composition are defined "implicitly," *i.e.*, as governing the transformations of the systems which they structure. [p. 10]

Organicism, as a structuralism, attempts to comprehend and transcend former dichotomies not by abolishing one of the poles but by linking them. The obvious examples in embryology are field–particle, structure–function, regulation–mosaicism, part–whole, and epigenesis–preformation. The link between the poles must be concrete to be valuable. It is insufficient merely to decree the old dualisms of biology to be resolved. Organization, laws of composition, and hierarchies constitute the subject of an organicist biology; the words are not explanations. It is commitment to this principle that differentiates "organic materialists" such as Needham from those still struggling on the fringes of the mechanism–vitalism paradigm such as J. S. Haldane or Lloyd Morgan.

The third defining characteristic of a structure is the power of self-regulation, which in turn implies conservation and a certain closure of the structure to the exterior. The "transformations inherent in a structure never lead beyond the system but always engender elements that belong to it and preserve its laws" (p. 14). The idea of closure or boundary means that in the process of development of an embryo from a state of lesser to greater complexity, the old limits are not abolished. The laws of substructures are conserved in the more complex whole. The elements of a structure are organized in their own right. Thus, the search for the unorganized starting point is meaningless. The process of integrating substructures demands the concept of hierarchy as part of the idea of regulation of form. Regulation, complexification, and boundry are closely interwoven.

In a chapter entitled "Physical and biological structures," Piaget discusses the function of his concept in two key natural sciences. For him the organism is the prototype of all structures, but a true organicism has only begun to develop after centuries of effort at reductionism in biology. Vitalisms have emphasized the notion of whole, but they do not qualify as structuralist perspectives, because their explanation of totality remained purely verbal. Piaget felt that Ludwig von Bertalanffy, inspired by the work of Gestalt configurations, was the first biologist seriously to explore the requirements of a structuralist organicism, which led to his "general systems theory."[20] The best example for Piaget of current structuralist perspectives is the work of Waddington, especially his idea of chreods. Waddington came to chreods from earlier thought on fields and problems of form.

So we have come full circle. This discussion on the elements of organicism began with form—the obsession of artists, poets, and biologists—and ends with form enriched by considerations drawn from chemistry, investigations into polarity of invertebrates, early field theory, and aspects of contemporary structuralism. But let us now look more closely at the foundations of the organismic paradigm in embryology. It is time to explore how Harrison transcended the limits of mechanism and how, avoiding any hint of vitalism, he set the problem of biological form in fresh perspective.

20. Paul Weiss in conversation said Bertalanffy owes his organicism to Weiss. They met in Vienna in 1922 and talked often about the notion of system and its possible applications. To see Weiss as a source of Bertalanffy's thought only reinforces this volume's contention that embryological work underlay the organicist paradigm for biology as a whole.

3

Ross G. Harrison

It has, therefore, been found advantageous to go to the lower vertebrates, particularly to the frogs and salamanders, for a material that may be obtained in abundance and which from the first is amenable to observation and experiment. That the amphibian mother casts her progeny loose at the time of fertilization, while not praiseworthy from the humane standpoint, is a boon to the embryologist.

Ross G. Harrison

A Pioneer in the Construction of an Organismic Paradigm

Ross Harrison's greatest contribution to experimental embryology might well be his insistence that the whole cannot be allowed to remain a mystery, penetrable only with the aid of mystical incantations. His contribution is so meaningful because he would not take the opposite course and deify analysis. Analytic methods had a purpose beyond themselves: to facilitate refocusing on the organism in all its richness. But in contrast to Needham and Weiss, Harrison, who virtually founded the science of experimental embryology in the United States, refused to be caught ofteñ philosophizing. In a sense it is strange to choose him as an ancestor of modern organicism. Nearly all his discourses on method lay initial stress on the need for analysis, on the responsibility to avoid teleological explanations. At first sight it would seem more sensible to look to Spemann as a cornerstone of organicism in his generation of embryologists. His concept of the organizer bordered on a deliberate use of psychological explanation in animal development. Spemann was hardly a vitalist in the sense of Driesch, but neither did the great German exercise the total discipline over his concepts of causality that Harrison did. However, it is precisely because Harrison so rigorously avoided vitalism or any related mysticism of the whole that his thought and experimental work are so important for the organismic paradigm. From his first work on the development of the fins of teleosts in 1894 to his last experimental paper on the suspected paracrystalline basis of symmetry in the amphibian limb rudiment in 1940, Harrison focused on the complex interactions of components in the animal system.

A useful way of exploring the philosophic and experimental under-pinnings of Harrison's work is first to look at the chronological progression of his interests, emphasizing their coherence and the embryological principles involved. Then a careful analysis of his methodological statements—especially on the part–whole problem, the legitimacy of the experimental method, and on the relation of structure and function in development—should prepare for a consideration of Harrison's treatment of field, gradient, and other organismic concepts. His examination of organization on the biological level drew him into molecular biology. It is well understood that bacteriological studies on the one hand and X-ray crystallography on the other led to the synthetic field of contemporary molecular biology. It is less well appreciated that Harrison's classic work on the foundations of symmetry and his conception of the structure of protoplasm constitute a third root, one nourished in the soil of a different paradigm. Finally, a close study of the Silliman Lectures, delivered in 1949 when Harrison was seventy-nine years old, should summarize his immense contribution to an organismic paradigm in embryology.

Harrison began his graduate work at Johns Hopkins under the tutelage of W. K. Brooks. Before receiving his Ph.D. in 1894, he spent more than a year working under Moritz Nussbaum in Bonn.[1] During this early period (1893–1895) Harrison's main interest was the development of the fins of teleosts. Within the context of that study he published on the mesodermal or ectodermal origin of bones. This work was relevant to his later study of the site and tissue of origin of the *Amblystoma* limb.

However, the major body of his work began in 1898 with the publication of his first experimental paper, whose topic was the growth and regeneration of the tail bud in frog larvae (1898). This paper marked the introduction of Born's method of transplantation into American

1. For biographical information on Harrison see especially Abercrombie 1961 and Nicholas 1961. Brooks was a major factor in the development of modern American biology. His students include E. B. Wilson, T. H. Morgan, E. G. Conklin. The nature of Brooks's influence on these extraordinarily creative men deserves serious attention.

embryology. In 1894 Professor Born of Breslau had observed in the context of his work on regeneration that pieces of frog embryos would rapidly heal together. It was possible literally to reassemble the parts of the embryo according to any pattern desired. It would be hard to imagine a better method to test the strength of the mechanistic paradigm. Throughout the first half of the twentieth century, transplantation techniques were essential to the testing and refinement of notions of regulation. Harrison quickly recognized the implications of the method, and in his desire to test the influence of the soma on the germ cells during development, he grafted the anterior half of one embryo onto the posterior half of another. He used two species with different pigmentation, so it was possible to follow in composite embryos the wandering and shifting of parts. It proved impossible to follow the original plan of testing the influence of somatic cells on reproductive cells. Instead, Harrison used his heteroplastic (derived from two species) combinations to study polarity of the amputated tail. He asked if the oral end of the tail rudiment were capable of regeneration and if so, to what extent. *Polarity*, when used by a morphologist, meant "not only symmetry, but also an internal cause for that symmetry, by virtue of which every particle of the organism has the same polar relations as the whole." It was well known that the posterior end of a cut tail could regenerate a functional organ. If true polarity reversal took place when the axis of the tail was reversed, it would imply that the inherent symmetry of the organism was extremely labile. Harrison found that the oral end could regenerate to some extent, but the character of the resulting organ was that of a trunk. If positioned favorably, the "trunk" could *function* as a tail, but there was no functional regulation such that the basic *structural* properties of the organism were rearranged. "Neither the present nor other experiments indicate that the influence of the organism as a whole upon the regenerating part is able to bring forth a heteromorphic structure, functionally adapted, out of material which would normally produce something else" (pp. 469, 481).

This first experimental paper shows Harrison's fundamental concern with symmetry and its relation to regulation. Use of the word *polarity* in organic systems implied the applicability of the analogy to the magnet. Harrison had limited use for the image because of its implication of forces of attraction and repulsion at the protoplasmic level. From his earliest work Harrison favored a structural basis for symmetry and was groping for the appropriate analogy. A simple machine analogy would not do, because it was incompatible with the regenerative and regulative phenomena of the organism. He recognized the relevance of functional regulation but rejected any conclusion that, in his experiments, "unusual relations imposed upon a regenerating part can call forth out of material which would normally be used otherwise, an entirely new heteromorphic structure, as a functional adaptation to new surroundings, or as the result of a striving to complete the mutilated organism" (p. 468). In sum, Harrison's first experimental work established the concerns and directions of his response which were to occupy him for the following forty years.

The next papers of Harrison that were critical to construction of an organismic paradigm concerned the development of the nervous system. In 1903 he published a study of the development of the lateral line system of amphibians. From this beautiful and complete investigation came the observation that the end of a nerve fiber connects early with its final site of attachment and then the nerve is drawn through the length of the body as the sensory epithelium extends. The observation was significant in his support of the neuron theory of nerve fiber growth. Then in 1904 he published a study of the relation of the nervous system to the developing musculature of the frog. The paper examined two important questions: (1) Was a stimulus from the nervous system necessary in order to start differentiation of striated muscle fibers, and (2) Were the normal processes of ontogeny regulated by functional stimuli? He placed young embryos with no differentiated muscle fibers into a chloroform–acetone (chloretone) mixture, which entirely inhibited action of nerve centers. Embryos raised in this medium immediately showed all the complex locomotory movements when they were allowed to recover. Harrison also removed the medullary tube (future spinal cord) from embryos and observed that good muscle fiber differentiation occurred in these animals without nerve fibers.

In this work Harrison gained insight into the relation of structure and function in the developing organism. Despite the fact that muscle fiber differentiation took place, some muscle atrophy was also observed in embryos without a nervous system. Both constructive and destructive influences were present. It was emphasized that the embryo was not just "a developing organism, in which the parts are important potentially, but also an organism which in each stage of development has

functions to perform that are important for that particular stage"
(1904a, p. 217). Roux had earlier suggested that development could
be divided into two periods, one of elaboration of structure and one of
functional development. The proposition was compatible with a strict
mechanism. Harrison stressed that his work showed considerable
overlap of the two periods even though the general distinction was
correct. He was, again, centrally interested in interactions of processes
and parts, even in the developing embryo. Nothing existed only for a
future use; the system had its present coherence. Otherwise it was too
easy to introduce either a teleological striving or a machine-like
placing of parts.

From 1904 to 1907 Harrison concentrated on the development of
nerve fiber. Operating from the perspective of the cell theory, and in
particular of the neuron as the source of fibers, he applied the experimental method to an area that had been the province of descriptive
labors. As Abercrombie noted in his biography of Harrison, there was
never any doubt in the embryologist's mind about the relevance of the
cell theory to the genesis of nerve fibers. Far from weakening his powers
of rational criticism and the search for a correct explanation, strong
allegiance to the theory gave Harrison a focus that is present in all
fundamental experimental endeavor.

The first answer given to the question of the origin of the nerve
fiber, which came from Schwann in 1893 and was supported by
Harrison's contemporary O. Schultze in 1905, stated that the fiber "is
a product of a chain of cells, which reaches all the way from the center
to the peripheral termination, these cells secreting the fibrillae within
their protoplasm much as an embryonic muscle cell secretes the contractile fibrillae" (1908b, p. 390). The opposing answer was that of
His (1886) and then Ramón y Cajal (1890), who held the nerve fiber
to be an extension of a single ganglion cell formed by growing out from
cell to periphery. It was impossible to decide definitively between the
two hypotheses, because the developing fiber in the normal embryo
was always found associated with spindle-shaped cells (Schwann cells
that form the sheath around a nerve). So in 1904 Harrison removed
the neural crest (area of the embryo alongside the medullary plate that
gives rise to the Schwann cells) from embryos of *Rana esculenta* and
observed that peripheral motor nerves developed anyway (1904b). The
fibers, traceable to the ventral area of the spinal cord and distally to the
normal muscle attachment sites, were naked, having been deprived

of the sheath cells. The next step in Harrison's argument involved removing the source of motor nerve fibers while leaving the neural crest in place. When the ventral half of the medullary plate, source of the ganglion cells of the motor nerves, was surgically cut out, no peripheral motor nerves developed. Therefore it appeared settled that the ganglion cell, not the Schwann cells, was the source of the nerve process.

The second pivotal question concerned the manner in which the connection between center and periphery was established, "whether there is a continuity *ab initio* (protoplasmic bridges) or whether the connection is secondarily brought about by outgrowth from the center towards the periphery." Harrison directed himself against the first view (Hensen's hypothesis, 1864), according to which protoplasmic connections remained between cells after division and "those that are used, *i.e.*, that function as conducting paths, persist and differentiate into nerves, the remainder disappearing" (1906, p. 128). The ganglion cell theory of origin did not deny the importance of the periphery, allowing it a possible role in guiding the growing process, but did exclude peripheral bridges giving rise to nerve fibers. Harrison's first experiments consisted in removing the center, that is, cutting out the medullary tube shortly after its closure. The result was total absence of peripheral nerves. The second tack involved altering the peripheral path. If the spinal cord were removed from a young embryo, a space was left above the notochord that filled with loose mesenchyme cells. After about a week, fibers arising from the brain were found growing posteriorly, extending as far into these abnormal surroundings as eight segments from the cut end of the neural tube. The third set of experiments involved transplanting pieces of the spinal cord to unusual surroundings, for example, under the skin of the abdominal wall. Small nerve trunks were found to develop from the transplants and to run for considerable lengths. One fiber stretched across the peritoneal cavity, having apparently made connection with its end organ before the separation of the splanchnopleure and somatopleure. This fiber ruled out entirely the action of any protoplasmic bridges. Harrison justly concluded from the three sets of experiments that the nerve center (ganglion cell) was the one necessary factor in the formation of the peripheral nerve.

With the above results firmly in hand, Harrison gave a complete response to the experiments of H. Braus, a supporter of the Hensen hypothesis. In contrast to earlier workers, Braus also believed that only experiment could solve the question of the origin of the nerve fiber. He performed a fundamental test that Harrison interpreted according to the neuron theory. Braus transplanted a nerveless limb from an embryo that had undergone the greater part of its development after having its spinal cord removed. Any protoplasmic bridges supposed to be originally present in such a limb must have degenerated because they were forced to remain functionless for a long period. If Hensen were correct, the source of fibers would have been removed. Braus placed the limb on the trunk region of a recipient animal and found that the extremity acquired a normal nerve complement distributed in the usual limb pattern. Braus had interpreted his experiments to be in accord with Hensen because he had not given proper consideration to the degeneration of any postulated pre-nervous, protoplasmic bridges. The real significance of Braus's work became apparent only in light of Harrison's results; that is, the structures contained within the limb must have had a critical importance in guiding the incoming nerve fibers, especially since even a nerve supply from an abnormal region was properly distributed. Branching could not possibly be determined by the ingrowing fibers alone. Further, lack of functional activity, either resulting from development in chloretone or placement of the transplant in an unusual position, did not interfere with normal nervous development.

The study of the entire question of nerve-fiber origin demonstrates several of Harrison's outstanding characteristics. From the start he was interested in the relation of structure and function and was not satisfied to accept as adequate a framework whose premises rested on paradigms from physiology (e.g., Hensen thesis). He approached each problem from as many perspectives as possible. His consuming focus was on *demonstrable* interrelations of parts of an embryo that had meaningful functions of its own but that was engaged in constructing a mature organism. Choice of the developing nervous system as the object of study enhanced intellectual concentration on problems of complex relationships; it was a system of integration par excellence. Maintenance of constant pattern in the face of unusual circumstances concerned him in its wider context of regulative phenomena based on the operation of relevant sectors of the system. Another significant Harrison trait is evident in the next bit of work he undertook: He sought an absolutely critical test of the neuron theory and in the process created the technique of tissue culture, inaugurating study of parts of the organism outside the body of the animal.

The crucial experiment involved two closely related tests. First, small pieces of clotted blood were introduced into the body of the embryo in the path of developing nerves. Not surprisingly, fibers were found in the clots. Then in the spring of 1907 Harrison's efforts to grow tissue completely outside the organism succeeded. (1907b). Pieces of tissue were taken from frog embryos at the stage immediately after closure of the medullary folds, that is before the differentiation of any nervous elements. The tissue was transferred to a drop of fresh frog lymph. The lymph clotted quickly, holding the tissue in place; in adaptation of a method from bacteriology, the preparation was sealed upside down over a depression slide. Normal development of form did not occur in the cultures, but individual tissue elements did differentiate into characteristic cell types. From medullary tube tissue, numerous fibers grew out, extending into the surrounding lymph clot. The highly branched ends of the fibers were observed to be quite actively engaged in a type of amoeboid movement. The result of the activity was that the protoplasm of the nerve cell was drawn out into a long hyaline thread closely resembling naked nerve fibers in the organism.

The first tissue culture experiment raised in acute form the problem of wholeness. Objections were made to Harrison that, at best, cells could only keep themselves alive in such an abnormal medium. The processes he observed had to be pathological and could not give important information about normal development. However, Harrison saw his work as a logical outgrowth from that of Driesch and Roux; he was testing powers of self-differentiation of parts. Driesch and Roux had been limited to studying germ cells and isolated blastomeres of the segmenting egg; Harrison extended the analysis to other cell types. The control, which assured him that he was looking at more than pathological reaction to disruption of the whole, was found in the differentiation in culture of muscle fibers from cells that would have given rise to such fibers in the animal. He also obtained in culture pigment cells and ectodermal structures such as the cuticular border and cilia (1912). Harrison was interested in any method, in this case tissue culture, that gave biologically important information. Exploitation of method for its own sake was not one of his sins. In addition to showing the extent of self-differentiation, culture systems allowed study of chemical and environmental factors upon differentiation of tissues.

But Harrison was primarily concerned with the application of tissue culture to morphogenetic problems. He recognized that because cell movement was a critical factor in the development of form it was essential to understand what factors controlled it. Nerve fibers never showed extension unless there was a solid substratum present. In the early cultures it was observed that cases where the lymph did not clot also did not result in fiber growth. Harrison carefully described the protoplasmic activity of the ends of fibers; movement always occurred along the fibrin threads (1910b). The shape of the nerve cells seemed to be influenced by mechanical tension in the clot, but tension did not account for the existence of cell movement. Extension of the fiber required endogenous cell activity. Direction appeared random as long as it followed a solid surface. In later work Harrison placed pieces of tissue in culture on a spider web frame and reported that extensions always followed either the web fibers or grew along the cover-glass surface (1914b). Fibers did not seem to exert either positive or negative chemotaxis on one another.

The foregoing observations led to the conclusion "that solid objects are an important and even necessary factor in the movement of embryonic cells." Harrison concluded that the reaction to solid surfaces constituted a true stereotropism and judged that there was no reason to suppose chemical stimuli were active in his experiments. If the parts of the nerve cells were differentially sensitive to surface contact, exposure to a solid surface would induce movement in a definite direction. In other words the cells were polarized and capable of responding to the tactile stimulus offered in the experiments. Barring previous regional differentiation in the cell, "the kind of reaction called forth by contact with a solid object could only be a clinging to that object or a recoil from it" (1914b, pp. 540, 542).

Harrison felt these results were significant for the understanding of normal processes.

> Since it has been shown that most embryonic cells are stereotropic, and that such arrangements as they assume in the embryo may often be induced under cultural conditions by reaction to solids, there is a presumption in favor of the view that this type of reaction is a potent factor in normal development also. Inferences as to what goes on in the embryo which are not based on exact information regarding the physiological properties of the tissue elements are

likely to prove erroneous. On the other hand, if we know the actual properties of individual cells in detail, it will be possible to form, on the basis of observation of normal development, an accurate conception of the influences actually at work in shaping the embryonic body. [1914b, p. 544]

Many incidences of cell movement occur in the embryo near the stage of development from which Harrison took his tissue. Cells of the ganglion crest migrate to many points. The lateral line rudiment shifts, in the course of several days, all the way from the head to the tail. Schwann cells move out along the nerve fiber. Cell movement is clearly involved in wound healing and nerve attachment to end organs, and paths of cell movement are a major factor in pattern determination. Showing nerve cells to be positively stereotropic in culture gave a clue to mechanisms of fiber distribution in the embryo. The hypothesis that fibers follow solid surfaces in the organism did not explain the specificity of final attachment to the end organ, but it did explain a good deal of nerve patterning without assuming special chemical differentiations or chemotaxis. Harrison speculated that final attachment might be analogous to attraction of egg and sperm and might resemble immunological processes. In sum, his work emphasized that it was possible to understand pattern formation even when it was as complex as the laying down of the nervous system.

In 1915 Harrison began a series of experiments that were to lead him him to fundamental conclusions on the nature of symmetry. From 1915 to 1925 he published a number of papers on the establishment of the principal axes around which the limb of *Amblystoma punctatum* developed. The experiments on limb laterality were originally suggested by work of Hans Spemann in 1910 and G. L. Streeter in 1907 on the amphibian ear vesicle. Spemann declared that an ear vesicle inverted 180 degrees developed in inverted position. Streeter found some normal development of inverted vesicles, but the regulation seemed to be due to rotation of the entire otic capsule. Both men worked on relatively late embryos, that is at a stage when the otic capsule had just closed. Harrison decided to examine the determinants of laterality in the limb system by using much younger specimens, that is at the stage of closure of the medullary folds. The general framework within which the work fell was that of determining the mode of representation of adult form characters in the germ. Most work on the question of preformation–epigenesis in the modern period had been done on the egg. Born's method of transplantation allowed Harrison to study the problem on an organ system after gastrulation.

Before he could undertake the main experimental analysis, it was necessary to determine precisely the area of the embryo destined to give rise to the limb. (Some early work in 1911 and 1912 had failed because regeneration from the host occurred. The investigator had failed to remove all prospective host limb tissue before placing his transplant.) Simple experiments located site of origin: extirpation of the body wall of the forelimb region, varying the size of the wound; extirpation of a specific portion of the limb region; removal of the limb rudiment and covering of the wound with ectoderm taken from another region of the embryo; removal of mesoderm alone, replacing the overlying ectoderm; removal of ectoderm alone, leaving the mesoderm intact; and fianally, transplantation of small masses of mesoderm from the limb region to beneath the skin on the embryo's side (1915). The results showed that the anterior limb bud was determined at the time of the experiments. The mesoderm of the region gave rise to a limb when transplanted to an abnormal site. Mesoderm, not ectoderm, was the critical germ layer in limb formation. And finally, the mesodermal cells of the region formed a clearly determined system as a whole, but all the cells were totipotent within the system, at least in forming muscle or skeleton. The exact area of the limb rudiment was not defined. Instead it was shown that the limb rudiment "many not be regarded as a definitely circumscribed area, like a stone in a mosaic, but as a center of differentiation in which the intensity of the process gradually diminishes as the distance from the center increases until it passes into an indifferent region" (1918, p. 456). There were several such centers of differentiation in the embryo, and their boundaries appeared to overlap one another.

In the course of demonstrating the field-like character of the limb bud, preliminary experiments showed the rudiment to be a harmonic equipotential system, a phrase introduced to embryology by Driesch to refer to a situation in which the potencies of all parts of the system were the same, the constituent cells being totipotent. Driesch felt that the existence of such systems was good evidence for an immaterial cause, the entelechy. Harrison explained such regulation in nonvitalistic, organis-

---

2. Harrison believed that the existence of a true equipotential system necessitated some sort

mic terms.[2] The experiments that demonstrated the character of the system were straightforward: extirpating half-buds and superimposing two buds. A whole developed from a part, and a single normal whole developed from two separate rudiments when fused together. With the limb system explored to a considerable degree of satisfaction, the main body of work on determinants of laterality could begin.

The experiments were designed to test whether the axes of symmetry were determined at the early stage under observation. The limb itself is asymmetrical, but the right and left members are mirror images of each other. At what time was laterality determined and what was the underlying cause? Three different circumstances relating to position in the embryo were taken into account: location, side, and orientation. A limb placed in its natural position in another embryo was said to be *orthotopic*. If it was placed in some other region (e.g., on the flank), the term used was *heterotopic*. Some limbs were grafted onto the same side of the body as that from which they came (homopleural), and some were placed on the opposite side (heteropleural). Finally, limb rudiments were placed either in upright position, with the dorsal border of the transplanted disk corresponding to the dorsal border of the wound (dorsodorsal), or inverted with the ventral border of the graft matched with the dorsal edge of the wound (dorsoventral). So there were eight possible combinations tested (1917). Each combination was observed several times and preliminary rules were drawn up to describe the results. The first rule stated that "a bud that is not inverted (dorsodorsal) retains its original laterality whether implanted on the same or on the opposite side of the body." The second rule was that "an inverted bud (dorsoventral) has its laterality reversed whether implanted on the same or opposite side." Third, "when double or twin limbs arise, the original one (the one first to begin its development) has its laterality fixed in accordance with the above rules, while the other is the mirror image of the first" (1917, p. 247). The last statement calls attention to the significant fact that the transplanted organs frequently reduplicated

---

of molecular hypothesis for the representation of adult form in the germ. Since the arrangements of the bud elements did not determine the final pattern, the final symmetry must depend upon properties of an intimate protoplasmic structure. It was here that the crystal analogy became central and here that Harrison was entering molecular biology. The crystal analogy was also suggestive of the design and logic of the limb laterality and symmetry experiments. Optically active asymmetrical molecular forms, such as D- or L-glucose, are mirror images of each other. But this simple basis was not the focus of Harrison's mature approach to the analogy. However, discussion of this topic will be more appropriate below (pp. 92 ff.).

themselves, forming double or even triple limbs with definite symmetry relations to each other. Often the redundant limbs were later resorbed and difficult to identify, but in early developmental stages they were quite definite. Possibilities for use of the crystal analogy are obvious.

Two of the four possible orthotopic combinations produced limbs that developed in normal orientation with respect to the cardinal points of the embryo: homopleural–dorsodorsal and heteropleural–dorso-ventral. These combinations were termed harmonic; the remaining combinations that showed reversed laterality were disharmonic. Harmony was a function not of a single variable but of both orientation and laterality. Harmonic combinations in orthotopic position yielded single, functional limbs (96 percent); disharmonic combinations most often resulted in reduplications (96 percent). In fact the original limb might be resorbed, leaving a functional mirror image of itself as the final product. It was important that the three rules of laterality led as often to disharmonic as to harmonic results. However, secondary factors, such as those that determined whether a twin limb would arise and those that produced resorption of the initial limb, resulted in adapted, correct appendages. Needless to add, Harrison was interested in understanding the mechanisms underlying the final adaptive result and felt no need to turn to vitalist categories such as striving.[3]

In the heterotopic group of experiments, where function was excluded, harmonic combinations yielded a large percentage of reduplications (54 percent). The disharmonic cases gave rise to single limbs 87 percent of the time. It seemed that with orthotopic grafts the dominant factor relating to twinning was harmony or disharmony of the combination. There was probably a tendency to reduplicate in all cases due first to the disturbance of the operation. Harrison explained the results by noting that the primary limb in a harmonic situation had the advantage of correct connections with the environment and so suppressed secondary buds. Reduplicating buds in disharmonic cases had the advantage of proper orientation and connection. The lack of special anatomical relations in the heterotopic class meant that reduplicated appendages in harmonic situations could not be suppressed. Left unexplained was the lack of twinning in disharmonic heterotopics.

---

3. Harrison's concern with regulation of both form and function is apparent. He concluded that both occurred, often hand in hand, but not necessarily. Functional regulation was largely dependent upon innervation. Form regulation was primary for harmonic combinations, but secondary (by rotation or reduplication) for disharmonic cases (see Harrison 1921a, p. 114).

But by itself it gave weak grounds for a classical teleological theory of development.

Of far more promise was the important analysis of form determination over time that Harrison was constructing. The general conclusion from the above experiments was that the anterioposterior axis was already determined at the time of transplantation. However, the dorsoventral axis was still either not set or reversibly determined.[4] Postulating that the intimate protoplasmic structure was the relevant level of the organism in the establishment of symmetry since any coarser grain was unable to harmonize with the demonstrated equipotential system, Harrison decided that the elements making up the cells of the limb bud could still be rearranged along one axis but not the other. Final orientation of the elements was not a function either of the limb by itself or of the surroundings, but of both together. This postulated interaction was a clear example of Harrison's use of organismic explanation. He was dissatisfied with both the machine analogy, which would have required that initial positioning of the cell parts decide the path of development, and with Driesch's radical conclusion that the fate of any part was alterable according to imposed new relations. The actual situation was more complex and required careful study of actual interactions and imaginative speculation about the required "grain of the mosaic."[5]

After completing the major part of the limb analysis, Harrison turned to another basic problem: growth regulation and coordinated growth of complex organs. For these experiments he returned to the method of heteroplastic grafting he had used in 1898. "Heteroplastic

4. In a later paper the effect of reversing the mediolateral axis was examined. It was discovered that the anterioposterior axis was determined first, then the dorsoventral, and finally the mediolateral. These experiments led to the final statement of the rules of laterality: (1) When the anterioposterior axis is reversed, the resulting limb is disharmonic. (2) When the anterioposterior axis is not reversed, the resulting limb is harmonic. (3) When double limbs arise, the original member has its asymmetry fixed in accordance to rules 1 or 2, while the secondary appendage is a mirror image of the primary one (see Harrison 1925b).

5. Harrison repeated his experiments on axes of symmetry of paired organs on two additional systems: the ear and the gill. The conclusions were essentially similar, but the gill, with its three-germ-layer structure, proved too complex to deal with adequately. In the ear the earliest operations (neurula stage) were performed before any of the three axes was established (complete isotropy). Then the anterioposterior, followed by dorsoventral and thirdly mediolateral, dimensions were determined. About the times of determination the organ rudiment was most likely to show developmental abnormalities, such as swelling distortions, as a result of experimental manipulation. See Harrison 1936a; refer also to Harrison 1921b.

grafting may be defined as the union of parts of organisms of different species into a single individual, or the combination of individuals of different species in double or multiple organisms living parabiotically."[6] Two organs were chosen for study: the limb and the eye. The study was initially suggested by the difference in the time of the forelimb's appearance in two species of salamander, *Amblystoma punctatum* Linn. and *A. tigrinum* Green. At the beginning of the larval period the limbs of *A. punctatum* were more developed anatomically and were fully functional, whereas the *tigrinum* forelimb of the same stage was still a nodule of mesenchyme without visible differentiation. But during the larval period, *tigrinum* limbs grew much faster, surpassing *punctatum* in size. By metamorphosis the latter limb was about half the size of the former. "The question arose, what would occur if the limb buds were interchanged before beginning their development. Would they adjust themselves to the new environment and develop at the tempo of the host, or would they maintain their own rate of growth and reach the ultimate size of their own species?"[7]

Owing to the mode of feeding, initial results were somewhat deceptive and led to postulation of an hormonal factor that would regulate growth in addition to internal constitutional factors of the limb tissue (1924). *Punctatum* grafts on *tigrinum* hosts were retarded in relation to the donor controls. These grafts not only grew more slowly than the normally fast-growing larval *tigrinum* limbs but also lagged behind the sister limbs still attached to their original bearers. The reciprocal experiments yielded comparable results: *tigrinum* grafts on *punctatum* were accelerated in growth relative to the remaining member of the donor pair. Nevertheless, graduate students of Harrison, Victor Twitty and Joseph Schwind, discovered that the retardations and accelerations were eliminated if the experimental animals were fed all they would eat—maximal feeding. Thus the circulating factor was reduced to "nutrient level," a slightly mysterious, but nonspecific parameter.[8]

Once the feeding problem was resolved, the general conclusion

6. Harrison 1935, pp. 116–57. Harrison worked on growth regulation from 1924 to about 1930, giving a major summary of the subject in his Second Harvey Lecture of 1933.

7. Second Harvey Lecture, reprinted in Harrison. 1969, p. 218.

8. Twitty's popular book *Of Scientists and Salamanders* gives a good account of the Yale "chief's" method of training his students and of the atmosphere of the Osborn Laboratory during his tenure. Harrison had many successful graduate students and definitely exercised a benign influence on their development. Their ranks include Samuel Detwiler, John Nicholas, Leon Stone, and Frank Swett.

from both limb and eye studies was unmistakable. The grafted organs grew at a rate determined by species-specific factors, unaffected by the host environment. But the situation was significantly different when components of the eye were combined—retina (optic cup) from one species and lens (overlying ectoderm) from the other. Here reciprocal size regulation occurred, producing an organ with the parts adapted in size to one another. Thus the *tigrinum* component grew relatively more slowly than usual and *punctatum*'s contribution speeded up its processes. The results held for both types of combination (1929). A further inter- action studied in these experiments was that between brain and eye. An eye larger than the normal host organ resulted in corresponding hyperplasia of the optic centers in the midbrain. The reciprocal again held. Optic nerves also were regulated, and frequently the experiments resulted in perfectly good, functional eyes.

The growth experiments marked a greater care on Harrison's part for quantitative sophistication in treatment of data. Using J. S. Huxley's formula for describing heterogonic growth systems, Harrison was able to obtain growth rate constants for the reciprocal experiments that were arithmetic reciprocals.[9] The purpose of making such calcula- tions was to attain a more exact expression of species-specific factors, which might in turn yield clues about underlying mechanisms and fruitful physical models. It is also obvious that the experiments repre- sent a sophisticated investigation on the organismic level. The sugges- tive model was the system with parts that influenced one another and were molded by the whole organism, not the machine with set parts and rhythms.

Another concrete example of investigation on the "biological level" lies in the work on the balancer and associated connective tissue formation, once again in the faithful newt (1925a). Balancers are rod- like appendages on the side of the head that hold the head off the stream bottom until forelegs develop. *Amblystoma punctatum* normally possesses a balancer whereas *A. tigrinum* does not. Transplanting the prospective balancer ectoderm onto a frog embryo (or onto a young *tigrinum*), Harrison found that the ectoderm was "capable of reacting with the mesenchymal ground substance of the latter, and transforming its outer layer into a balancer membrane, as it does normally with

---

9. The formula is $y = bx^k$, where y is the magnitude of one part at a given point in time, x that of the other part, and k the constant ratio between the growth rates of the two, found by deter- mining the slope of the line given by plotting x against y on a double log graph.

tissues of its own species" (p. 409). The experiment showed that appropriately localized tissues even from different groups of animals could
interact to produce a functional organ.

The balancer region is a system similar to the prospective limb or ear
areas; that is at some point during gastrulation organ-forming potencies
seem to be localized.

> During this period the areas that are to give rise to gills, balancer,
> nose, ear, other placodes, hypophysis, and the lens are segregated
> according to a pattern, not, however, with any very definite bound-
> aries of its several components, but rather in a manner that the
> organs just enumerated appear as centers of differentiation, with
> their respective potencies most intensely active at certain points
> from which the intensity gradually diminishes peripherally.
> [p. 410]

Area boundaries overlap, and tissue of an intermediate region is
organized into one organ or another as a function of the center whose
influence predominates. Such systems came to be called fields, but it is
not a word used by Harrison in that context until the late 1930s. As
Waddington cautioned later, the term *field* should convey more than a
geographical meaning; he suggested a term such as *area* or *district* when
one does not intend to refer to the complex of processes involved in
organ formation (1956, p. 23). Harrison's discussion of structures and
processes involved in axis determination of the limb and ear *is* an
analysis of the nature of a field and constitutes one of the first and most
basic of such studies. Harrison did not use the word *field* very often and
especially not as a deliberate theoretical concept as Weiss would have
done; but nonetheless, it was his fundamental work that first gave
concrete content to the organicist notion.[10]

Study of the balancer led to important observations from three
additional perspectives, one of which linked Harrison to the later con-

---

10. In his Second Silliman Lecture, "The egg and early stages of development," Harrison
discussed the definition and properties of fields. Using the typical analogy of a magnetic field of
force, he summarized Weiss's concept as a "center of activity or of differentiation from which
a characteristic quality diminishes gradually toward the periphery of the area." If the field center
were removed, neighboring parts assumed its character and function. Fields of similar character
could be fused or halved and regulation would ensue. Fields have individual natures (limb, ear,
and so on) and gradually become divided into specialized subfields. The basis of these entities
was probably a repeat pattern of a structured protoplasm, which is the form the crystal analogy
finally took for Harrison.

cerns of Weiss (connective tissue development). First, not only was there differentiation in space but also in time. The specific ectoderm was competent to differentiate into a balancer only within certain temporal limits. Second, Harrison described the spatial and temporal connections of balancer development with nerve, circulatory, and skeletal components. That analysis is an apt example of his appreciation of complex interconnection of structures and processes. Finally he made a cogent analysis of connective tissue elaboration, in particular, of the laying down of the balancer's basement membrane. The membrane was formed from condensation of the intercellular "ground substance" in the mesenchymal region underlying the evaginating balancer epithelium. The cellular elements of the mesenchyme did not participate directly in formation of the connective tissue structure. The original diffuse matrix material was changed into a closely patterned mat of reticulum fibers. Factors in the condensation could not have been strictly mechanical, since no basement membrane formed underneath adjoining structures undergoing similar evagination movements. "We must look to some other kind of activity in the epithelial cells, and one naturally thinks of an enzyme action which condenses or coagulates the underlying diffuse intercellular ground substance transforming it into a fibrillar tissue which gives almost the same chemical reactions as reticulum" (1925a, p. 412). The suggestion of enzyme involvement in form development was a fertile one for the organicist resolution of the structure–function polarity.

The last major experimental paper of Harrison was written a year after his retirement from Yale in collaboration with a pioneer of protein crystallography, W. T. Astbury of the Textile Physics Laboratory at Leeds (Harrison, Astbury, and Rudall 1940). The paper is a gold mine of forward-looking speculation and attempts at experimental demonstration. The work involved taking X-ray diffraction photographs of several living embryonic tissues from chick and newt: neural plate, neural tube, ear ectoderm, notochord, and yolk. It was hoped the photographs would support the molecular orientation theory of tissue polarization.

> For some time past, evidence has been accumulating, mainly from transplantation experiments, that certain embryonic systems are at first isotropic with respect to their future differentiation and only gradually become oriented and polarized. This secondary condi-

tion has no immediate outward expression, and since the systems in question are known to be equipotential, the changes observed must be based upon some finer structure of protoplasm, which is probably of a molecular order of magnitude. [p. 339]

In the case of tissue that was still isotropic, any molecular elements responsible for polarization would not yet be oriented. Molecular re-arrangement at the time of polarization might be detectable by X-ray crystallography, but technical difficulties prevented a clear answer. The photos did not show any definite orientation but gave only a ring pattern characteristic of a disoriented protein. The results were not taken as refutation of the hypothesis, because of the difficulty of detect-ing a postulated, oriented, noncrystalline array of globular molecules in living tissue. It was extremely difficult to study protein structure even with true crystals. Detection of a "paracrystalline" state, that is, a con-dition in which the elements had freedom of movement along one or more axes, was exceedingly unlikely. It was a significant victory simply to get X-ray pictures from living material. The basic conception under-lying the trial remains potentially valid, and perhaps a contemporary repeat of the work would be successful.

A second important method was applied to embryological problems in the 1940 paper: optical examination with a polarizing microscope. Orientation in biological tissue had been studied before with polarized light (Schmidt 1924). Birefringent material was seen in Harrison's material, especially at cell membranes. Harrison noted that their work was preliminary and should be followed up systematically. "Especially should the cell boundaries be examined thoroughly, for it is there, perhaps more than anywhere else in the cell, that we may expect to find the seat of directive forces" (Harrison, Astbury, and Rudall 1940, p. 355). A glance at current journals in cell and developmental biology reveals the appropriateness of the admonition to study cell membrane systems in relation to form problems.

With an overview of Harrison's life work in mind, it is possible to evaluate his philosophy of method as he developed it early in his career. One's approach to method implies a good deal about one's particular view of the part–whole relationship. Harrison never de-viated from his assertions that the experimental approach was appro-priate and necessary in the study of animal development. This commit-

ment was central to the founding of the *Journal of Experimental Zoology* in
1903.

> It was a group [the founders and contributors to the journal in its
> early years] with varied interests but with the common conviction
> that the application of radical experimental methods was feasible
> in zoology and other descriptive sciences, and that only through
> this course could the biological sciences expect to approach the
> exactness and systematic consistency of the physical sciences.
> [1945, p. xiii]

In the context of defending tissue culture as an avenue of understanding
normal processes of development, Harrison set forth his general position. All vital processes were associated with "the complex things we
call organisms." Any disturbance of the whole, no matter how slight,
constituted an introduction of abnormal conditions and might be
eliciting unsuspected regulatory phenomena. Arguments against experimental manipulation in embryology must be applied to the simplest
operation in physiology too, and even to experiments of physics and
chemistry. Regulatory phenomena in organisms were only an especially
complex instance of the interaction of large numbers of causes in all
natural systems. No natural system is simple in the classical mechanist
sense. The proper conclusion would be that experimental analysis is
difficult and full of pitfalls for the unwary, not that true understanding
cannot be gleaned from the operations. Processes of analysis were the
means to resolve normal phenomena into more elemental factors,
"from which, for purposes of verification, phenomena like the original
may be recomposed or be represented more or less perfectly by some
kind of model, according to the completeness of the knowledge gained
by the analysis" (1912, p. 184).

The whole, then, must never become a fetish; analysis should be
pushed to its limit. The abnormal and altered were pregnant with clues
to normal processes; to ignore such sources of information would be to
refuse to concretize concepts of form in embryology. Organization and
wholeness for Harrison were not answers to biological questions; they
were the biological questions par excellence. The crux of his analytical
approach lay in his insistence that analysis was performed in order to
allow refocusing on the whole organism, on its problems of integration.
His own use of a given method was always to ask a question of the

organism, never to exploit a tool of analysis for its own sake. He initiated a method—tissue culture—so central to the functioning of modern biology that it is nearly impossible to list its applications. But Harrison, not interested in pursuing culture techniques, returned to the organism and continued to probe it for replies to very well put queries.

Biological explanation for Harrison was a roundabout process. There were no criteria that assured certainty or unqualified application of experimental results to natural processes of development. The best check of applicability lay in "careful comparison of what occurs in experiments with what can be observed in the normal developing organism" (p. 185). In general, comparison was a process appropriate to analogical reasoning. Careful comparison allowed one "with a varying degree of probability to draw conclusions regarding the causal nexus of the factors within the normal body" (p. 187). Harrison cited Ernst Mach in support of the importance of a comparative approach.[11] Comparative and analogical procedures were suitable for more than traditional classification and morphological study. They were basic to explanation and complementary to experimental analysis. Causal relations were revealed by analysis; appropriate questions and final refocusing were arrived at by analogy.

Harrison drew on J. S. Mill for his notions of "causal nexus" and "plurality of causes." He followed Mill in believing that full explanation of development would come only with synthesis of organisms from simple known constituents. However, synthesis could be made at "different stages of the analysis with components of greater or lesser complexity" (1912, p. 185). It was not necessary to resolve the whole into ultimate atomic units. Units themselves, Harrison implied, were of greater or lesser complexity. He never talked in terms of total reductionism. The most direct statement of Harrison's position came in the 1917 address to the American Association of Anatomists.

> We must resolve the organism into elemental structures and processes, and make new combinations, to find out how the factors bear upon one another. ... When pushed further, the experimental methods of study will enable us to state the facts of morphogenesis in simple terms of cellular activity, and we may hope to

11. Harrison 1917, p. 409. Mach delivered an address in 1894 entitled "On the principle of comparison in physics," in which he showed how the concept of potential had led to linking previously dissimilar concepts such as pressure, temperature, and electromagnetic force.

connect these with the results of microchemistry in localizing intracellular activities, and ultimately identify problems of structures and functions with those of the protein molecule in its manifold physico-chemical relations. [1917, pp. 407–408]

Even at the last stage the crucial problem was organization and interaction of the protein molecules.

But although Harrison was not a doctrinaire reductionist in his philosophical opinions, he tended more in that direction than either Needham or Weiss, who talked much more explicitly in terms of the fundamental relevance of levels and hierarchy. The difference is more apparent than real in that Harrison had an indisputable appreciation of investigation on the biological level in its own right. Nevertheless, it is largely because of his lack of explicit development of the idea of hierarchy that Harrison is seen in this book as a pioneer in the formulation of an organismic paradigm rather than as a full adherent. He manifested the ambivalent traits that Kuhn saw as peculiar to such pioneers: retaining parts of a philosophy of explanation more appropriate to a strict mechanism while laying the groundwork for an approach (a good theory of hierarchy) that transcended the machine framework. Experiment was all too new in embryology in the first decades of this century for Harrison to be interested in modifying the dictates of thorough analysis. Experimental method and the machine paradigm are by no means inseparable, and Harrison was not operating out of exclusively mechanistic presuppositions.

Regulatory phenomena and form problems comprised the core of Harrison's experimental and theoretical concerns. He has been described as a father of nonvitalist organicism in this volume because of his relentless attention to organismic questions and because of a rejection of facile oversimplification while stressing experiment. In particular it is important to recognize his work on growth regulation, patterning in the nervous system, interactions in the formation of intercellular connective tissue, and analysis of asymmetry and field organization. In keeping with Kuhn's description of the process of paradigm change, Harrison realized fully the strains in the machine analogy and pushed his own experimental work beyond the boundaries of its explanatory power. Harrison was also linked to the nascent organismic paradigm community. The link was less in the sense of close-working groups, such as that around the technical and theoretical advances of crystallographical analysis of biological molecules in England, than in the sense of sharing emerging new metaphors and expectations.

The clearest statement of his adherence to an organicist perspective was made in a speech delivered in 1932 on the inadequacy of the concept of determination in development (1933). He began with a reference to the weakening of concepts of causality in contemporary physics. But just as physicists were exploring new frameworks of explanation, biologists were dogmatically pushing ideas of strict causal determinism. "It is as if a sort of Presbyterian biology were coming upon the scene just a physics is about to go over to the Baptists" (p. 306). The concept of determination in embryology was related to the epigenesis–preformation controversy. Harrison's position on determination was illustrative of the organicist transcendence of that controversy.

Both the preformationist and epigeneticist arguments implied that adult characters were in some sense *implied* in the egg, but preformationism took the further step of postulating that all the parts of the organism were actually *contained* in the germ. Embryology had no note of substantive history or novelty, but Harrison emphasized that the term *determination* (*Bestimmung*) as Roux used it in the 1880s was not meant in a strict preformationist sense. The term was meant to apply to localization of parts in the germ with reference to their future disposition. In 1932 Harrison cited approvingly the 1902 definition of determination given by E. Korschelt and K. Heider:

> We count under this rubric the whole cycle of questions that deal with the disposition of constituent parts of the embryo with reference to their future fate. Accordingly, it has to do with the origin, nature, and localization of organ-forming factors—a field that embraces the fundamental questions of embryology and although already taken up from various sides, one that still remains very much in the dark, [p. 307]

The inadequacies of the basic concept and an exposition of an alternative formulation of the problem made up the remainder of the speech.

In describing events of differentiation that occur after a certain amount of initial segregation of substances has taken place the egg, the term *determination* had a certain legitimacy. It referred to Roux's questions about dependent versus self-differentiation. But biologists were not satisfied with this general use of the concept, and they attempted to find the exact cause and time of determination of a primordium to form one and only one end organ. As Harrison observed,

> *It might all be well enough if we confined our use of "determination" to the processes themselves,* and described the changes that take place as differentiation proceeds, but *trouble begins when,* as is more frequently done, *we use the word to denote a state* and ask the question whether an organ rudiment is "determined" or not, meaning thereby whether it is so fixed as to its capacities that it can do but the one thing that it does do. [p. 308 (italics added)]

He went on to explain that experiments revealed no single criterion of fixation. Quite the contrary, "one could not fail to conclude that the isolated part tends to form a greater variety of structures than when left in place in the embryo" (p. 311). Parts of the organism showed embarrassing plasticity.

Even the strict segregation pattern in the mosaic eggs of ascidians, which seemed so intimately related to strict determination of a region's fate, was of only temporary significance. Adult ascidians showed powers of regeneration and developmental plasticity that defied inclusion in any concept of determination. Attempts to include such phenomena under the strict mechanist category led to an endless search for "neoblast" or reserve cells, which were never "determined" but lay hiding among differentiated cells, jealously guarding their totipotency.

Experiments on the optic-cup–lens system delivered the final blow to the idea of determination for Harrison. In particular, W. Le Cron had demonstrated that if the optic vesicle were removed from *A. punctatum* embryos immediately after closure of the neural folds, the overlying ectoderm did not develop into a lens, as it would have done with the optic cup in place. However, the same ectoderm transplanted to the ear or heart region did develop into a good lens. Which structure determined which? Harrison's conclusion was that "the emphasis upon 'determiner' and 'determined' leads to a very lopsided and often erroneous view of the process, for *it is questionable whether one factor can influence another without itself being changed*" (p. 315 [italics added]). Emphasis on such interrelations was fundamental to the organicist perspective on the part–whole problem.

In the same speech the Yale embryologist related Spemann's organizer to the problem of determination and expressed his dissatisfaction with certain implications of the notion of an organizer. Harrison's views here are critical to the assertion that he struck roots of a true organicism whereas Spemann, accepting the limiting assumptions of the mechanistic paradigm, hinted at vitalistic categories of explanation (Hamburger 1969). The most exciting single event of developmental biology in the twentieth century before Watson and Crick revealed the structure of DNA was Spemann's discovery of the organization center and organizer in the amphibian egg. Traceable to the gray crescent of the egg, the center turned under at gastrulation to form the roof of the primitive gut. Its powers included the ability to mould the whole embryonic axis and to fix the various regions of the future nervous system. Any preconceived notions of preformation and fixity of germ layers degenerated in the scramble to uncover the nature of this remarkable embryonic region. But Harrison was among those who cautioned early that the material upon which the organizer exerted its influence was already highly organized. "The organizer, itself a complex system with different regional capacities, merely activates or releases certain possible qualities which the material acted upon already possesses. The orderly arrangement which results depends not only upon the topography of the organizer but also upon that of the system with which it reacts" (1933, p. 317). For Harrison interaction of parts meant the processes that bound complex systems to one another through time, each system affecting the other within the whole organism.

In another context Harrison revealed what he meant by calling the organizer a "complex system." The organizer showed "marked regional differences. A regionally differentiated organizer acts upon a less differentiated material. Both have something to say as to what will be formed." Furthermore, the observed regional specificity could not be ascribed to a simple activity gradient but had to rest upon structural characteristics. Harrison suspected that the organization center, like the limb region, owed its asymmetry to field factors. "I cannot agree with Dr. Wright on the origin of gradients. It seems to me that we must postulate a primary polarization of structural units, and that this involves cytoplasm as well as nucleus. ... The matter of asymmetry is part of the same problem as polarity."[12] And the organizer was an instance of asymmetrical organization.

Harrison summed up his position on the organizer and the determination concept by stressing that successful explanation in embryo-

12. Remarks are taken from Harrison's discussion notes of Sewall Wright's 1934 lecture on genetics of growth anomalies of the guinea pig. The notes may be found in box 12, 1933–36, folder 2, of the Harrison files in Sterling Library Archives at Yale.

logy had to be measured by "simplicity, precision, and completeness of our descriptions rather than by a specious facility in ascribing causes to particular events" (1933, p. 319). He presents his own synthetic theory of development in a 1936 lecture (1937).[13] This theory constituted the essential link between Needham and Harrison in the sense of a paradigm community, just as the frame for viewing the patterning of the nervous system tied him to Weiss. The fundamental notion was "to refer the changes in the developing organism to the conditions imposed by the configuration of the protein molecule and its accompanying chemical and physical activities" (1937, p. 372). The colloid theory of the nature of protoplasm was replaced with an appreciation of intermediate crystalline structure. Protoplasm was seen as more than a gell of substances; pattern was essential.[14]

Harrison speculated that primary polarization of egg arose from alignment of the protein molecules oriented as a function of their dipole character. The opposite chemical properties of the two poles would result in different chemical reactions and electrophoretic transport of charged molecules to different sectors of the egg. Field properties would be set up by forces arising from the chemical structure of the cell, and material gradients could be one expression of the situation.[15] Substances produced under direction of the genes would be localized in the structured cytoplasmic milieu, resulting in different chemical reactions

13. The remarks in this article are a condensation of the Harvard Tercentenary Lecture, which will be discussed fully below.

14. A colleague of Harrison at Yale, George Baitsell, delivered a paper in 1938 at the AAAS meetings on "A modern concept of the cell as a structural unit," in which he clearly described the concept of structured cytoplasm. Applying modified notions of crystallinity to cytoplasm helped bridge the gap between ideas of organic and inorganic nature and led to concrete pictures of linked scales of complexity. Baitsell's paper reflected the benign influence of Harrison in these areas of thought. The paper was an advance announcement of molecular biology, that is, a "clear view of the elemental patterns of protoplasm" (see Baitsell 1940, p. 6). Baitsell may have been the first to use the term *molecular biology* in a public paper. Jane Oppenheimer notes that Astbury called himself a molecular bioligist in 1939, but I am aware of no earlier use of the expression (see Astbury 1939, p. 125; also see Oppenheimer 1966, p. 12). The recent and indispensable history of molecular biology is Olby 1974.

15. Harrison wrote that Conklin, Morgan, and Spemann advocated a molecular basis for the fundamental principle of vital organization. Driesch too referred relations of symmetry of the organism to symmetrical relations of the intimate protoplasmic structure. Child, on the other hand, thought of functional (metabolic) properties as the basis of axial differentiation and gradients. Harrison criticized Child, noting that "such gradients may well be an expression of the polarity rather than its cause" (1921a, p. 92). In any event Harrison was opposed to the kind of structure–function dichotomy that Child embraced.

taking place in various regions. New local centers of activity with a
potential to differentiate into subfields were thus established. Side
chains of the oriented protein molecules were envisioned as the locus of
specific chemical activity (an intimation of proteins functioning simultaneously as enzymes and structural units), and realtive reaction velo-
cities would account for greater and greater local diversity of action. As
the egg continued to divide, the above processes accounted for accompanying local diversification of cells. But each cell of an organism would
retain a characteristic cytoplasmic asymmetry within which gene-
directed metabolic processes occurred. The idea that each cell contained the full genetic endowment was broadened to include the possession also of a basic cytoplasmic structure. Within this framework,
differentiation, dedifferentiation, and determination took place. There
was no need to postulate neoblasts, any more than there was a need to
search for the irreversibly determined, differentiated cell. No elements
of the cell—genetic, metabolic, or cytoplasmic—were conceived as
either inactive or unstructured.

Significant cell movements such as gastrulation and neurulation were
explained by cell-shape changes due to the action of crystallization
forces resulting from changes in molecular configurations during
chemical reactions.[16] "Differentiations are in a sense, then, the by-
products of cytoplasmic activity and are accompanied by movements
involving change of form" (1937, p. 373). At no point in the scheme
does a single cause determine a single effect; systems of oriented
processes differentiate into subsystems coordinated by their mutual
functioning. Many lines of Harrison's bold theory remain unconfirmed,
but his approach still constitutes perhaps the richest contribution to a
coherent theory of development. The concept of fields resulting from
structured activity is a typical organicist resolution of the field–particle
polarity. The resolution rests, essentially, on going beyond structure–
function dichotomies.

The fundamental organizing insight in Harrison's approach to
development was his conception of the role of protein molecules. Proteins were important because they gave him a hold on a source of asymmetry of the desired "grain." "The existence of the equipotential system
necessitates, in fact, the assumption of some sort of molecular hypothesis

16. The recent demonstration that microtubules and microfilaments involved in cell-shape
changes are necessary for the folding of the neural plate to occur in *Xenopus* embryos is ample
confirmation of Harrison's speculations (see Karfunkel 1971).

for the representation of adult form in the germ. . . . In other words, it is the intimate protoplasmic structure that underlies symmetry" (1921*a*, pp. 87–88). For his conception of the role of proteins, he was indebted particularly to W. T. Astbury, Dorothy Wrinch, and Joseph Needham.

The latter two were associated through the Theoretical Biology Club. The forms of intellectual interaction among these biologists were typical of a paradigm community. As Eugene Hess observed recently, "An indispensable condition for development of molecular biology was the recognition that biological structures are organized on a molecular basis" (1969, p. 668). All four individuals were essential to the fulfillment of that condition.

Astbury was responsible for valuable early X-ray analyses of crystalline protein structure. The first major solution of the structure of a biological molecule came only in 1925, when O. L. Sponsler deciphered the cellulose fiber. His method was applied to silk protein (fibroin) by H. Mark about 1929. Astbury himself worked on textile fibers, and it was to him that Harrison turned for collaboration in the search for oriented crystal structures in living tissue.

Dorothy Wrinch was interested in applying a gemetrical approach to the problem of protein structure. Seeing the need to exploit such methods as chemistry, geometry, topology, crystallography, and physical chemistry, she proposed a type of closed fabric structure for proteins based on a cyclol ring form (1938). She was eventually shown to be wrong about the linkages in proteins—they are essentially long chains, with the amino acids joined by peptide bonds, folded into characteristic shapes. But her theoretical work functioned as a positive stimulation to men such as Harrison and Needham. From the beginning Harrison felt her work was related to his own search.[17]

Joseph Needham discussed his conception of role of liquid crystals in protoplasm in his Yale Terry Lectures of March 15, 18, and 19, 1935. The correspondance between Harrison and Needham before those lectures, and then afterword about the book *Order and Life* based on the lectures, reveals the intellectual relationship between the two men. In a letter dated January 11, 1937, Harrison indicated to Needham how much he had drawn on his conception of a paracrystalline organization of protoplasm.

17. In a letter dated December 30, 1937, Harrison indicated to Dr. Wrinch his desire for her help in his own speculation. See Sterling Library Archives on Harrison, box 24.

For my Harvard address [the Harvard Tercentenary of 1936], I drew very heavily on the literature you refer to in the third lecture ["The hierarchical continuity of biological order"]. ... I am afraid some of my friends think I have gone 'nuts,' as we say here, on the subject of protein molecules and the paracrystalline state. I tried a few X-ray diffraction pictures of the developing embryo last spring, but so far with negative results. One will need the collaboration of a first-rate physicist, familiar with the field, to accomplish anything and I hope to interest someone of this description in the work.[18]

Needham, in his turn, wrote in 1935 that he considered Harrison to be his mentor and guide at Yale, so much so that he had considered moving from Cambridge to New Haven to pursue his work on chemical embryology. Harrison felt that Needham's efforts to unify concepts of biochemistry and morphogenesis were extremely important.[19]

Although a generation older, Harrison himself was not the least active of the four workers listed above in laying the foundations for an organicist molecular biology. He began thinking in molecular terms very early (at least by 1921) and built molecular models in his Osborn laboratory constantly. He was influenced by H. Prizbram, who referred symmetry and polarity relations of organisms to the arrangement of particles in a space lattice. However, Prizbram had little appreciation of an organicist approach, and Harrison's originality resided in his use of the crystal analogy within such a perspective, with a full "realization how vastly more complicated these relations are in organisms than in crystals."[20]

It is instructive to look with care at the precise way Harrison developed the crystal analogy in his own work. Axial differentiation in the embryo could be compared to spatial relations of atom groups in certain carbon compounds. At the center of a tetrahedron, by analogy, one could assume a carbon atom linked to the four groups occupying the angles of the figure.

By hypothesis the groups at the angles are supposed to be at first all

18. Sterling Archives, box 32.

19. See Harrison's letter to Lancelot Hogben about Needham in support of Needham's candidacy for the Royal Society, box 31, folder 3, dated January 6, 1939.

20. Harrison 1925a, p. 499 (see also Prizbram 1906). Harrison also drew from such workers as R. S. Lillie, who as early as 1919 wrote a theoretical analysis of the crystal analogy in which he treated organisms as bounded, structured processes (see Lillie and Johnston 1919).

alike. If one of them should be changed by some reaction, the structure of the molecule would become polarized, and if all the molecules should assume approximately the same orientation, the system which they constitute would show a similar polarity. If two of the groups become differently modified, then the structure becomes bilaterally symmetrical. And, finally, if three become modified, so that all four are different, then the arrangement becomes asymmetrical as in the case of optically active substances with an asymmetric carbon atom. In the last phase there are two kinds of individuals, which are exactly alike in every respect, except that they are mirror images of one another. [1921a, pp. 88–89]

The experiments on the limb and ear lent themselves to this analogy readily. Some kind of paracrystalline organization, specific for a type of cytoplasm, would underlie form relations and form changes—morphology and morphogenesis. Progressive orientation of protoplasmic elements (restriction of degrees of freedom) could account for polarity and symmetry, without any need to postulate the cell as a homogeneous system. Crystal organization in organisms was itself an example of an intermediate level of organization, joining processes of organic and inorganic nature. And perhaps most significantly, Harrison's use of crystal analogies allowed him to bypass assumptions of the mosaic–mechanistic theories of development about part–whole relations and to account for the existence of equipotential systems without turning to either entelechies or classical machines.

Harrison's life work was beautifully summarized in a series of lectures he delivered at seventy-nine. The six Silliman Lectures of 1949 were entitled "Organization and development of the embryo." There is no better way to tie together this consideration of Harrison as a pioneer of organicism in contemporary developmental biology than to follow him through those lectures and the papers he relied on in their preparation. The concerns, the theoretical expositions, and the experiments speak for themselves.[21]

21. The complete Silliman Lecture notes are unpublished. I am indebted to Sally Wilens, long-time research associate of Harrison, and to the archive section of Sterling Memorial Library for xerox copies of the lectures. All quotations from the lectures come from this source. The book edited by Wilens, *Organization and Development of the Embryo*, cited earlier, contains the papers Harrison most relied on in composing his talks. The bulk of the supporting material in this book has not been taken from these papers, but from less readily available material in order to complement what Wilens has made so easily accessible. (Hereafter Sillman Lecture notes are cited in text as SL.)

The Silliman Lectures

> Though we think of it as a thing, the organism is really, as has been
> aptly said, an event in space-time.

In his introductory lecture of the Silliman series, Harrison observed
that development from egg to adult is an intimate personal experience
for each of us. The importance, fascination, and mystery of embryology
spring from this source, just as our physical involvement in organic
evolution gives this other historical branch of biology its unique place in
the history of ideas. The first lecture sets forth Harrison's position on the
nature of organization and the problem of levels in biology. Starting
from a bare dictionary definition, he emphasized two aspects of organization: configuration and relationship. He noted that all science deals
with organization and that in biology the concept is relevant on several
levels, each composed of units from a lower rung. The simplest units
exhibiting the biological level of organization are cells, which are, of
course, heterogeneous themselves. "The continuity between generations being through the germ cells—cellular organization must be taken
as the starting point of any account of the developing creature. Then
the organism, even the most complicated, *is* the cell, in the configuration and function of which the whole mature organism is implied"
(SL 1, p. 10). At the other end of the biological scale are societies of
organisms. Whatever the position on the scale, it is essential to study
both constituent parts and their relations to the whole, but all philosophical approaches to biology, from the most mechanistic to radical
vitalism, have admitted these commonplaces. The crux of the issue is
the nature of the units: Is the search for the ultimate uncomposed unit
justified?

Harrison's clear response in *no*. Cells are thoroughly heterogeneous;
"but it is not merely the presence of all these things (nucleus, cytoplasm,
molecular aggregates, micelles, etc.) that enables the cell to live and to
function. They must be there in proper spatial relations; hence the
emphasis on configuration." Even the atom itself, he emphasizes, "is
resolved into a constellation of particles having a characteristic configuration for each element" (p. 3). With the vanquished conception of
an ultimate simple atom, the view of arrangement of parts dictated by
the machine analogy also breaks down. How then are the levels of the
organism related to one another?

Harrison rejects the two vitalistic resolutions of the problem of hierarchy: the theory of emergence of Lloyd Morgan and the holism of General Smuts. Concentration on emergence had "interposed unnecessary obstacles in the way of our investigation." It was never evident how various degrees of organization emerged, and special acts of creation were, he alleged, strongly implicated.

> It is asserted that the entities occupying each level have properties peculiar to that level, which are not deducible or predictable from the properties of the units of the lower level. ... But it is an advance in our knowledge of water to know that it is a compound of oxygen and hydrogen and it may be said of hydrogen that along with its molecular weight, another of its properties is that under certain conditions it combines with oxygen to form water.

Holism was guilty of obscuring the idea of the whole instead of seeing unity as the fundamental question open to experimental analysis. "Its is impossible to develop science wholly from the top down or from the bottom up. The investigator enters where he can gain a foothold by whatever means may be available" (p. 4).

The correct approach, then, to configuration is to concentrate upon the organization proper to each level. This course implies an appreciation of indeterminacy in biology. No two biological units are ever exactly alike. Not only must the biologist use the tools of statistics, he must also realize he faces difficulties analogous to those of contemporary quantum physics. Experimental procedures alter the very unit being observed. And finally, the biologist must allow for different time scales appropriate to each level of organization. The rhythms of physiology, development, and evolution cannot be reduced to a homogeneous measure of time. The biologist must avoid the fallacy of misplaced concreteness, or else he is blind to the "problems of organized complexity" with which he must deal. Harrison here has implied that biology, as well as physcis, must surrender the mechanistic dream. Both have to confront the implications of indeterminacy, quantum phenomena, and relativity. The proper view of relations among levels of organization is indicated by the term *integrative level*. The aim of science must be "to scale them," not to homogenize them (pp. 4–7).

In the remainder of his first lecture and in the second talk, "The egg and early stages of development," Harrison described the early work in embryology and discussed concepts of normal development, egg polarity, the Roux–Driesch controversy, fields, and organizers. His positions were drawn from the papers analyzed in earlier sections of this essay. In the third lecture he returned to a subject whose study he had made possible, "The autonomy and dependence of cells and tissues in development." This lecture was a contemporary meditation on the cell theory that had been so fundamental to Harrison's study of isolated cells outside the body. Harrison described the history of the study of cell autonomy and placed the work in the context "of the antithesis which . . . originally led to much controversy which is not by any means settled: whether the organism consists of a large number of individual units or cells or whether it is consolidated into a whole, which has more than the combined capability of its constituents" (SL 3, p. 1).

After acknowledging the early work on blood cells and the always central contribution of Roux, who introduced the concept of self-arrangement (*Selbstordnung*), Harrison related the factors in his invention of tissue culture. His observations on the differentiation of various cell types in culture, as a test of Roux's formulation of self *versus* dependent differentiation, led to his critique of the determination concept. Describing the morphology and dynamics of cells in culture, Harrison stressed the basic point that cultures themselves were "organized" in the strict sense of the term. The old dichotomies of autonomous parts *versus* strict dependence on the whole were inappropriate. To further develop this point, Harrison reviewed both the work of Holtfreter on ectoderm and endoderm combinations and tissue affinity and other studies on axial or spherical organization of tissue masses in culture. "Here we have the borderline between the primitive organization of a tissue culture and the higher organization of an individual" (p. 7).

Harrison concluded the first half of the lecture by summarizing the considerable achievements of tissue culture up to 1949—which included demonstration of unlimited capacity of growth and reproduction in many cell strains, marked powers of differentiation of many tissues in nongrowth media, proof of the neuron concept, study of cell movement and aggregation—and by stressing the need for continued study along the fertile lines opened up. The latter half of the lecture was taken up by discussion of H. V. Wilson's sponge disaggregation work, mosaic cleavage and regeneration in ascidians, degeneration and regeneration in hydroids, slime mold morphogenesis, and pigment-cell development. All these systems provide rewarding tests of relative cell autonomy and clues to understanding the organism's "organized complexity." An example of Harrison's intellectual position is his conclusion to the section on slime molds: "These mycetozoa ... bring out in a more striking way the contrast between the cell as a unit or individual and the cell as part of a unit of higher order. These two roles alternate. The cells when free constitute an 'equipotential system' according to Driesch's definition and the part that each plays in constituting the whole is a function of its position" (p. 18). Such phenomena were crucial for an organicist, but nonvitalist, theory of development.

In the fourth lecture Harrison turned to the nervous system, a topic he stayed close to throughout his career and one that represents the most significant link between him and Paul Weiss.[22] The Silliman speaker described the embryogenesis of the nervous system in detail, emphasizing its complexity and the plethora of unsolved problems. He warned of the limits of such analogies as the telephone system, declaring that specificity and irritability of the nervous system were too fundamental for the image to provide much insight. He described with care his work from 1904 to 1910 on the origin of nerve fibers. Within that context he went on to evaluate various theories of nerve connection and growth such as neurotropism, chemotropism, and stereotropism. He cited Weiss's experiments with directed frameworks and rectangular and triangular frames, which had confirmed that nerves follow a directed course during development.

Another Weiss contribution mentioned in this lecture was the experiment of constricting a regenerating nerve fiber and observing the damming of material coming down the central axon stump. The work emphasized the metabolically active nature of the nerve cell as a whole and the close connection of cell body and extension. The morphological conclusion of Harrison in 1907 was thus extended to physiology: The nerve cell body was beyond doubt the source of the axon.

In the last sections of the lecture the speaker treated the problems of selectivity in nervous connection, the correlation of structure and

22. Ross Harrison first invited Weiss to come to Yale to work in 1928. Weiss reported in an interview on July 22, 1970, that his wife's parents were opposed to the couple's move at that time. But in 1931 a Sterling fellowship was arranged for Weiss and he arrived that year at the Osborn Laboratories, where he immediately set up a tissue culture laboratory. Harrison had abandoned the technique years earlier. Weiss conducted his important studies (two-center experiment) on stereotropism as an influence in pattern formation in nerve and fibroblast cultures while at Yale. Weiss and Harrison were never close working partners, but they were very sympathetic to each other and their relationship continued after Weiss went to Chicago in 1933. The paradigm community relationship between the two biologists will be considered more fully in the chapter on Weiss.

function during embryogenesis, form and function regulation in the spinal cord and brain, and regeneration. He displayed an obvious familiarity with an extensive literature on the nervous system. His contribution consisted in the integration of this material into a provocative portrayal of the questions answered so far and those remaining to perplex the modern worker. What he did not know then was that the recent work on optic tectum–retina connections was to be a fundamental investigation of axes and polarity (field relations), as well as of the nature of neural specificity between fiber and end organ. Both areas were of immense concern to Harrison.

The fifth lecture, "The symmetry of organisms," was based on the 1936 Harvard Tercentenary Lecture. The essential problem, however, was not true symmetrical organization but residual asymmetry of organisms; it was this study that occupied so much of Harrison's attention. In the speech Harrison explained that symmetry comes from commensurability and implies order, regularity, and arrangement. Geometrically symmetry is defined by operations of rotation, inversion, and translation. In nature, crystals and organisms embody the rules of symmetry; this simple fact underlies the historical analogy between crystal and organism. Harrison's work may be seen as a search for the appropriate degree and nature of the analogy in modern embryology. In our period, attention has been focused on internal laws of order for both sorts of entities; external form is a function of principles of arrangement, of inner patterning.

In the lecture Harrison reflected on the discovery of optical isomers by Pasteur in 1848. The discovery of molecular asymmetry had been a principal turning point in the relation of chemistry to biology. Optical isomerism provided Harrison with the analogy for his own version of the organism–crystal relationship. But it was clear from work on coiling in snails that molecules with the same asymmetry could produce organisms with opposite, mirror-image symmetry. Therefore it was too simple to postulate a one-to-one relationship between molecular pattern and protoplasmic structure. The clue to the dilemma lay in the suspected presence of a special type of crystal organization in organisms: liquid crystals. Such labile structures may change their orientation. "They are, in other words, para-crystalline and are often fixed in one or two dimensions instead of all three." In this context Harrison interpreted his work on the axes of symmetry in limb, ear, and gill systems of the newt. Molecular models showing successive substitution of four groups bound to a central carbon atom, initially very suggestive, were inadequate to the complexity of the organism. Rather, "the model showing progressive orientation of asymmetric molecules will explain the facts better." It further gave a means of understanding twinning across reflecting planes, a perplexing phenomenon encountered continually in the course of limb and ear experiments. "Twin crystals are very common and in cases of asymmetric forms, they frequently are the mirror image of each other. . . . This phenomena [*sic*] then speaks very strongly for the crystalline or paracrystalline nature of the living tissue making up the ear vesicle" (SL 5, pp. 3, 8, 7).

Harrison concluded his important observations with a simple but far-reaching statement.

> The significance of all this detail, which I fear may have bored you, is that it gives crucial evidence that these two quite different systems, the ear and the forelimb, are made up of units arranged in a repeat pattern which becomes definitely more and more oriented. In this respect they are similar to the egg. . . . In fact, that kind of organization seems to pervade all living matter and will have to be reckoned with in any theory of the organism. [pp. 10–11]

In the last lecture, "Development and growth in complex systems," the limitations of the classical crystal analogy, rather than the power of the organicist version, were explored. Crystals grow by accretion, and addition to each axis is proportional to axial relations of the lattice. "Growth of organisms is more complex, since they grow internally and are made up of many different components with different rates of increase" (SL 6, p. 1). D'Arcy Thompson was the first to analyze differential body proportions by referring them to a Cartesian coordinate system and applying rules of transformation. Different shapes were derived from a common form. Similar relationships among forms had long been appreciated by artists, and Harrison cited Albrecht Dürer's *Treatise on Proportion* as an example. The union of organic and artistic form underlies the perspective of the lecture.

The content of the paper was drawn from studies on chimeras, organisms constructed of parts from different species. Such work traces back to the first embryonic transplantations of Gustav Born about 1890. Harrison sketched his experiments on heteroplastic transplantations. He included his own and others' studies of limb, eye, gills, and heart, trying to sort out problems of form and function regulation and species-specific rates of growth.

The general conclusion to the Silliman Lectures is reprinted in full in

Wilens's text. The substance is that there are two basic levels of organization in biology, the cell and the individual, which meet in the organization of the egg. In that sense, embryology is the most fundamental discipline of the life sciences. Since "each and every living being can be encompassed in the organization of a single cell of its species" the problem of the embryologist would be simple if classical preformationist tenets were valid. But in the early 1890s Driesch exploded one version of the mechanist's dream and underlined the cardinal problem of development: form regulation. Harrison would not accept Driesch's solution. Focusing instead on regional differentiation in the egg, he elaborated an organicist theory of development: The organism contains a microstructure with an oriented and polarized repeat pattern. "In other words, the egg and early embryo consist of fields—gradients or differentiation centers in which the specific properties drop off in intensity as the distance from the field center increases, but in which any part within limits may represent any other." Dependent differentiation or induction involves two fields, "each with its intensity gradients, thresholds of activity and sensitivity, and each with time limits on its function" (1969, pp. 258, 260, 261). The organization of the elements of a field explains regulation within boundaries. These simple building blocks are precisely the ones common to Harrison, Needham, and Weiss.

4

Joseph Needham

Organization palpably appears at all size levels. Form is no longer the perquisite of the morphologist, and molecular exactitude no longer the preserve of the chemist. If I thought like this in 1935, I am even more convinced of it in 1967; the bridge is almost built.

Joseph Needham, 1968

Biology is largely the exploration of fibre properties.

Joseph Needham, 1935

A Great Amphibian

From his earliest years Joseph Needham (b. 1900) felt himself drawn to appreciate and comprehend antithetical modes of human experience in philosophy, science, religion, and culture. It is not surprising to find such a person examining the polarities of field and particle in the embryology of the 1930s. The organismic paradigm was woven from many threads; it required the convergence of disparate disciplines, nationalities, and philosophies of science. If Ross Harrison manifests the contribution to an organismic paradigm made by the American school of experiemental embryology, with a huge debt to the Germans, Needham embodies the currents of British developmental biology, again with significant links to Germany. Needham, who saw as his task the construction of a bridge between biochemistry and morphogenesis, was well suited for his role in a decisive period in the history of biology.

Trained in biochemistry at Cambridge in the 1920s, Needham was strongly indebted to Fredrick Gowland Hopkins, the founder of biochemistry at Cambridge. Hopkins, who is best remembered for his work on the structure of tryptophan and for the discovery of glutathion, continually stressed the need to appreciate the chemical *geography* of the cell.[1] He did not directly focus on form problems in ontogenesis, but he encouraged such an intellectual disposition in his students. Needham recalled that his mentor was by 1896 keenly aware of the need for work on development of the chemistry of the egg. About 1921 Needham himself was attracted to what he later called chemical embryology when he chanced upon a 1914 dissertation by Klein that demonstrated a change in inisotol concentration in the hen's egg during development. After his dissertation work on inisotol, finished in 1923, Needham applied himself to a variety of problems in the biochemistry of development until the early 1930s, when he began to focus on the chemical nature of the amphibian organizer. The years leading up to that work show an extremely interesting intellectual and experimental development culminating in a nonvitalist organicism. Attention to Needham's intellectual history is particularly rewarding because he so openly acknowledged and struggled with the strains of the mechanist–vitalist paradigm. A critical turning point in his own thinking occured in the early 1930s, a time that also saw the founding of the Theoretical Biological Club, a group extremely important to the articulation of the new paradigm.

It would be useful to examine Needham's experiments in two phases, from 1923 to 1934 and from 1934 to 1944. Highlighting the transition between the two periods are the studies of Hans Spemann and his collaborators in Freiburg and the truly impressive investigation of development by Holtfreter in Berlin-Dahlem. With an adequate appreciation of Needham's experimental concerns, one must then turn to their philosophical context.

From the mid-1920s until about 1931 and the publication of *The Great Amphibian*, Needham was occupied with an analysis of the history of vitalism and mechanism and a justification of his own neomechanism. Beginning with his acquaintance with Joseph Woodger and the ensuing discussions at the Woodgery on theoretical biology, Needham developed his mature position on organicism. Of foremost importance

---

1. Hopkins coined an aphorism that pointedly conveys the heart of his vision: "Life is a dynamic equilibrium in a polyphasic system." His work derived from that of W. B. Hardy, who studied structure in colloidal systems. Needham considered Hardy a pioneer in building a bridge "between the largest organic molecules and the smallest intracellular structures" (see Needham 1936, pp. 130–32; see also Hardy 1899). For a good view of Needham's debt to Hopkins, see his 1962 paper entitled "Frederick Gowland Hopkins" (*Perspect. Biol. Med.* 6: 2–47). See also Price (1973) for a provocative summary relating Needham's history and training to his later interests in the history of Chinese science.

in his reevaluation of scientific and philosophic matters was an introduction to Marxism and his subsequent political development. It would be profitable to gauge the influence of his political world view on the construction of the organismic paradigm. Finally, a consideration in depth of *Order and Life*, the Terry Lectures of 1935 published in 1936, should summarize and focus Needham's positions on form, organization, fields, particles (fibres and crystals), and hierarchical levels—the critical elements of organicism. *Biochemistry and Morphogenesis* will also be profitably explored in this section on Needham's speculative contributions to biology. A brief coda exploring Needham's post-World War II perspectives and opinions on developmental biology will complete the examination of his role in the new paradigm's formation.

Needham's introduction to the chemistry of ontogenesis resulted in his early publications of 1923 and 1924 on inisotol, which offered methods of quantitating its concentration in the avian egg, problems of synthesis in the animal body, and metabolic behavior in the developing egg (1923, 1924). This research was quickly followed by a variety of investigations of chemical processes in marine and avian eggs. Using microinjection techniques, he studied hydrogen ion concentration and oxidation–reduction potential of marine material (1926*b*). Attention was turned early to energy sources in ontogenesis, resulting in studies of nitrogen and carbohydrate metabolism in embryos (1927). The goal of providing a full chemical description of development unified all these investigations. Serious effort was made to relate the work to evolutionary history of the organisms, to questions of embryonic function at various points in development, and finally to an overall ground plan of animal growth. In the years before 1934 Needham did not yet have a single experimental focus for the unification of form and biochemistry, but he was groping in that direction through the more purely chemical study. The strand of developmental mechanics, or experimental morphology, which was to be such a critical component of his final synthesis, was not present in Needham's own work until 1933–34. Nevertheless, three major papers before that time are worth considering in detail in order to discern the workings of the mechanistic framework, its gradual disintegration, and its transformation into an organismic perspective. These papers are also important in allowing insight into Needham's constant early efforts to treat the embryo as a complex whole. It is precisely this commitment that later led him to an organismic paradigm. The early work prepared the ground; the later involvements introduced the twin notions of hierarchy and field that took Needham beyond concern for neomechanism and neovitalism.

First, studies on nitrogen metabolism directed him to a consideration of "The biochemical aspect of the recapitulation theory" (1930a). Ernst Haeckel's principle of recapitulation, summed up in the aphorism "ontogeny recapitulates phylogeny," represented an effort to explain embryological form solely by reference to adult morphology. Embryos were thinly disguised replicas of successive evolutionary stages. This type of explanation was formally idealistic, and Needham was seeking a mechanistic description of embryogenesis. He saw himself in the tradition of Wilhelm His, who had attempted to introduce physical explanations into embryology in the late nineteenth century and to work out the mechanics of development. Needham wished to probe the power of chemical explanation in an area given to formal analysis of heredity. Many phenomena in the embryo, such as the *foie transitoire* discovered by Claude Bernard, could be understood as significant transitory stages with definite functional relevance to the developing organism. However, there remained phenomena for which no clear, independent function could be assigned and which seemed to support the recapitulation principle.

Needham described in detail one such example, the nitrogen metabolism sequence of the chick, and demonstrated that only a strict causal explanation permitted a coherent understanding of the events. In the initial portion of its development the chick excretes about 90 percent of its nitrogen as ammonia, then as urea, and finally as uric acid. Marine invertebrates excrete their nitrogen as ammonia, fish and amphibians as urea, and the saurian branch of the reptiles and birds as uric acid. One possible alternative to the recapitulation principle in such cases was to postulate that an earlier state acted as a formative stimulus for the subsequent mechanism, but the ammonia–urea–uric acid series did not easily lend itself to that explanation. Needham felt it was more convincing to interpret the sequence as relating to a gradual increase in the organism's complexity. Thus, a kind of recapitulation theory was retained in the form of development from simple to complex, and from that point of view it would be legitimate to compare ancestral and embryological forms. The analogy would stress transitions and lead the investigator to search out the mechanisms involved; it would not be an explanation in itself as Haeckel's analogy was. So "embryos only recapitulate what they must, and in a word, recapitulation is itself explained by the physico-chemical requirements of the developing organism" (p. 156). In the revised principle the formative action of an earlier state in relation to the later condition would be a subset of the general category of increasing complexity. In sum,

> the fertilized egg cell ... would not profitably be regarded as a recapitulation of the protozoan ancestor ... , but nevertheless there *is* an analogy, and in the same way it may be held that the ammonia–urea–uric acid sequence occurs in ontogeny simply for the same reason it occurred in phylogeny, *i.e.*, because it is a transition from the more simple to the more complex. The reason why the chick does not excrete uric acid from the very beginning would, therefore, be that it was not until a certain point developed in the machinery for doing so, not that a urea stage was essential phylogenetically. [p. 151]

Needham went on to discuss other events in development, such as appearance of hormones, from this point of view. He attached significance to two additional examples: acquisition of the ability to maintain the constancy of the internal environment and the increase of energetic efficiency during development. Needham made modest experimental contributions in both areas. (See, e.g., 1926a, 1933c, 1933a.) The critical point is his integration of experimental concerns into his broad synthetic goal: a chemical understanding of embryogenesis under the organizing principle of increasing complexity and integration. It was to this point that the organismic paradigm would speak. But Needham employed the machine analogy first: "The tendency would now be to regard the developing embryo as an exceedingly complicated machine, in which there are no idling wheels and layshafts, although no doubt all the mechanisms are not in gear at the same time" (1930a, p. 149). He was never to abandon use of the machine metaphor, but its use was significantly different in his later concerns.

Needham elaborated his image of idling wheels and layshafts in a paper entitled "On the dissociability of the fundamental processes in ontogenesis" (1933b). Like Harrison, the Cambridge biochemist refused to let appreciation of the wholeness of the organism become an excuse for avoiding rigorous causal analysis. In this paper he was concerned to show the extent to which processes normally integrated

in the embryo could function autonomously, that is, processes could
be thrown out of gear with one another. The most appropriate metaphor here was without doubt the machine, with all its implications
for the part–whole issue in biology.

> It is already clear that embryonic growth can be stopped without
> abolishing embryonic respiration, and conversely, it is probable
> that growth or differentiation, under certain conditions, may
> proceed in the absence of the normal respiratory processes. There
> are many instances where growth and differentiation are separ-
> able. It is as if either of these processes can be thrown out of gear
> at will, so that, although the mechanisms are still intact, one or
> the other of them is acting as "layshaft" or, in engineering terms,
> is idling. [p. 181]

He followed this use of an engineering analogy with the caution that
attention devoted to a breakdown of integration is justified by the goal
of understanding the "means whereby in the normal embryo the
fundamental processes are integrated." The paper surveys a broad
selection of the biological literature and touches on the employment
of a great variety of techniques. The work unites them all by an explicit
insistence that the unity of the embryo is not a mystical absolute but
can be understood by attention to the organization of distinct processes.
The synthetic approach taken by Needham in this paper is typical.
Most of the work discussed in it was done by others, but he performed
the service of focusing the implications with the assistance of a powerful
metaphor.

Needham used metaphor in a manner that conforms to the requirements outlined on pp. 9–12 above. Explanation implies a picture, and
analogy is a vehicle for connecting the internal subjective perception
of the structure of a phenomenon with the public function of theory
building.

> Previous experiences spring to mind when an analogy is put
> forward, and the art of choosing an analogy consists in making
> sure that these psychological overtones will as far as possible
> correspond with the relevant elements of the analogue. And, above
> all, in certain circumstances an analogy may provide a framework
> or net of co-ordinates, in which a previously inchoate mass of
> information may advantageously be assembled. [p. 210]

There are at least three interesting examples of the image of "disengagement" that prompted Needham to ask further questions about the picture he was drawing. First, closely associated with the idea of gears is the notion of reversibility. He discussed this implication in the context of work on differentiation and regression in planaria and in sponges. Under conditions of starvation, planaria can reduce markedly in size without changing morphologically. But in ascidian regression, considerable dedifferentiation accompanies loss of mass. Experiments on sponge disassociation and reassociation focus on a similar problem, but it remains unclear to what extent reversals in growth and differentiation are involved. The point at issue here is that the metaphor Needham chose caused him to assemble a great deal of material that might otherwise have appeared unrelated.

The second example is Needham's search for a "primary shaft" in development. He had distinguished two types of dependence on a whole: existential dependence, in which a part would cease to exist if separated from the whole, and dependence with regard to properties, in which certain aspects of isolated parts are modified. The latter was indicated by analysis of the relevant literature; there were definite boundaries to the independence of parts, definite selectivity in the engagement and disengagement of gears. "It is as if each fundamental process represented a layshaft which may or may not be in gear with the primary shaft, and the animal economy is obviously so constituted that more than one secondary gear can be engaged with the primary shaft at one time." Within a context of substantial autonomy of processes and systems, the metaphor required one to search for a principal axis. Needham felt that the primary shaft could not be identified with any single chemical reaction, but had to consist of a complex of reactions that could provide the organism with a minimum amount of energy to maintain its integrity or organization in the physical world. He settled on basal metabolism as the "primary shaft, or rather, the automotive unit to which the primary gearshaft is attached" (p. 211).

However, identification of a principal axis only leads one to ask with more intensity about the *manner* of engagement or integration. This question illustrates the third example of following out the implications of the machine analogy. This query about the nature of organization drew Needham beyond the limits of the very metaphor that necessitated the inquiry.

> The difficulties of imagination are here acute, but it is perhaps
> easier to form some idea of how the synthetic processes of growth
> engage with the maintenance metabolism, than it is to picture the
> engagement of differentiation. . . . But in speaking of differentia-
> tion we enter a world remote from chemical conceptions, a world
> of form, a world of "organising relations above the molecular
> level," the nature of which we do not understand, and the ter-
> minology for which has not been invented. [p. 212]

The key problem lay in understanding the principles of organization
in even the simplest biological systems. Until some hint of these laws of
integration was uncovered, it was impossible to speak of increases or
decreases in organization. Like Harrison and Weiss, Needham looked
to the idea of structure, a primary organismic notion, for a solution.
Structure was not a static scaffolding but rather a condition maintained
by active metabolism. Work by Vles and Gex in the late 1920s had
shown that the absorption spectrum for cytoplasm was not characteristic for proteins until after cytolysis. This result was taken as evidence
for a special dynamic structural state of living protoplasm. Again in
concert with Harrison and Weiss, Needham scanned the work on
protein structure for further guidance. He felt the work of Astbury
would be of the greatest importance to embryology since it revealed
the fiber patterns of the protoplasmic fabric.

Via the proteins Needham was led to assess complex cytoplasmic
interactions between very large molecules. In the last year of the
nineteenth century Needham's teacher, Hopkins, had battled the
concept of the biogen molecule, a postulated giant entity supposed to
account for all the mysteries of life. Hopkins had felt that the idea
obscured quite answerable questions by substituting a vague dream.
Needham's criticism of the senior Haldane's treatment of organization
was similar, but Needham insisted strongly that the proteins merited
a different status than the biogen molecules.

> But if we are driven to take into account the forces which operate
> between molecular aggregates, it will only be because the facts
> imperatively demand it, demonstrating as they do the existence
> of organising relations in the living cell above the highest limit of
> complication expressible in terms of organic chemistry. And the
> recognition of the cell as a unit of enormous internal organization
> would not be, like the biogen-molecule theory, a portmanteau

explanation discouraging research, but a form of description with physico-chemical meaning, not supra-chemical in the Drieschian sense, because of the presence of an immaterial organising agent, but supra-chemical in the sense of J. H. Woodger and L. J. Henderson, because of the presence of inter-molecular forces and relations never seen at any lower level of organization. [p. 213]

The third paper of Needham's early experimental period relevant to his role in building an organismic paradigm is entitled "Chemical heterogony and the ground-plan of animal growth" (1934b).[2] If the publication on autonomy of processes propelled Needham beyond the limits of the machine paradigm via the idea of levels of organization, this work placed him firmly in an organismic framework via the notion of field. D'Arcy Thompson had done the first significant work on biological fields through his use of transforming relations displayed on Cartesian coordinate systems. A simple extension of his insight had been accomplished in the analysis of heterogonic growth, that is, differential growth of parts of an organism.[3]

Needham wished to extend the idea of a common ground plan of growth, with basic mathematical relations describing seemingly widely divergent forms of growth, to the chemical realm. "And just as we think of organs or structures as parts of a morphological totality, so we may think of substances or groups of substances as part of a chemical totality." By abstracting from time, morphological form, and absolute concentrations of chemical substances, Needham was left with a series of ratios corresponding to the relative values of chemicals during comparable stages of development in different groups of animals such as crustaceans and mammals. He considered seventeen items such as water, glycogen, nonprotein nitrogen, and sulfatides and concluded that "organisms of extremely different morphological form give identical differential ratios for a given chemical substance" (1934b, pp. 81,

2. This paper represents Needham's most mature treatment of a topic he first considered some years earlier. In each case in this book I have chosen as the principal reference the latest expression of a theme for a particular period of development of Needham's thought because he often published several times on similar issues. In a letter to Woodger dated September 26, 1932, Needham said Julian Huxley's recent book had "fired me with the idea of charting all the sets of data we possess on change in chemical constitution of embryonic body with age on double log paper, and I find that the ideas of his on heterogony are quite applicable to 'growth' of individual chemical constituents such as glycogen or fat."

3. The formula developed in 1924 by Julian Huxley, $y = bx^k$, has already been discussed in the chapter on Harrison.

104). So there existed some sort of "unitary ground-plan of animal growth" deformable in space–time analogous to the shapes of D'Arcy Thompson. Needham did not follow up on this very general work, but the fact that he was drawn to it indicates his tendency to seek organismic, nonvitalist explanations of biological phenomena. He was more prone to seek answers in complex systems of processes related by field laws than to postulate single key chemical reactions as simple, unitary causes of subsequent events.

Before describing the events surrounding the discovery of the amphibian organizer that were to be so important for Needham's experimental and philosophical development, it would be enlightening to glance at a monumental work he accomplished by his thirty-first birthday, the three-volume *Chemical Embryology* (1931).[4] The body of the text is a compilation of virtually everything known at the time about the chemistry of ontogenesis. The overall purpose was to lay the foundation for a chemical understanding of form; that is, to unite biochemistry and Entwicklungsmechanik, eventually seen as a task within an organismic paradigm. Its contents were elaborations of positions Needham had reached before he focused on the chemistry of the organizer; the above three papers adequately cover the essence of those concerns. The text included ample sections on the unfertilized egg as a physicochemical system; growth; increase in complexity and organization; respiration and energetics; carbohydrate, lipid, and protein metabolism; enzymes, hormones, and vitamins; and immunology, as well as treatments of the biochemistry of egg, fetal membranes, and placenta. But *Chemical Embryology* contained in addition prolegomena and a theory of chemical embryology written about 1928 and epilegomena, written in 1931, that highlight the subtle switches of concerns as Needham began to operate from a strict organismic perspective.[5]

4. Part 2 of volume 1 contained a 160-page history of embryology from a chemical standpoint. This section was later published as a separate book (see 1934a). A second revised edition was printed in 1959. The text illustrates Needham's propensity to reinterpret the history of science from the perspective of postmechanistic Western frameworks. His efforts beginning in the 1940s, which have resulted in the publication of four of seven planned volumes entitled *Science and Civilization in China*, express the same goals. The analogies between organismic philosophies of the East and West are probed for their relation to science and technology.

5. In a letter to Joseph Woodger dated February 1, 1930, Needham discussed the change in his own perspective from the writing of the first and last parts of *Chemical Embryology*. Woodger had found the introduction philosophically unsatisfactory. Needham wrote in response, "It is not really satisfactory to me either. It was written at the outset of writing the book, *i.e.*, nearly two years ago, and therefore at a time when I was much more impressed by the arguments of

The introductory sections of his book stressed a vision of science committed to the program of Galileo: "To measure all things that can be measured, and to make measurable what cannot yet be measured." Needham agreed with T. H. Huxley's words that the goal of biology was to deduce the facts of morphology from "the laws of the molecular forces of matter" (1931, p. 9). This was the mechanistic idea of the primacy of function.

> It seems always to have two meanings, firstly, the Epicurean-Lucretian one which Huxley adopts here and Roux so brilliantly developed, in which shape is regarded as the outward and visible sign of properties of matter itself, and secondly, the Aristotelian one . . . in which psychical factors are introduced as the essential elements in the ultimate analysis of shape.[6]

Needham followed his statement of allegiance to an essentially corpuscularian philosophy with a description of his neomechanism, which

the old-fashioned vitalists than I am now. I felt then that my particular line of work needed a defense but I feel now, as you do, that criticism rather than defense is what it needs. . . . It may be instructive for readers to notice the subtle change in point of view which will appear when the epilogomena are compared with the introduction." Woodger's critique went very deep, for he believed that the *metaphysical* claims not just the methodological ones of mechanism had to be taken seriously and transcended. The letter from Woodger to Needham dated January 25, 1930, contains Woodger's remarks on the subject. They curiously reject Kant and Whitehead at the same time. In particular he felt Whitehead was most helpful in his pre-*Science and the Modern World* days, when his work was "of more restricted scope." Perhaps the most relevant remarks in the long January letter concerned Woodger's criticism of the mechanistic search for simple causes. Woodger had begun to appreciate the power of explanation in terms of pattern and organization. He believed "current concepts of physics and chemistry are very abstract from the standpoint of organized entities. . . . Even biology (to its shame) has not found adequate concepts for dealing with what is characteristic of biological organization. . . . Hence I do not think it is sufficient to say that the difference between living and non-living organisms is 'a quantitative one, expressible in degrees of organization [Needham's 1930 belief].' The important point is to study the different possible *types* of organization. Crystals and organisms . . . both exhibit the type of order I call 'hierarchical' but they exhibit it in very different ways which can hardly be accurately called difference of degree." And finally, "Knowledge requires to have a structure which reflects the structure of fact and to be adequate, its structure has to be of the same degree of manifoldness as that of the fact."
I am indebted to Dr. Needham for copies of and permission to use these letters.
6. Ibid. There is some irony in citing T. H. Huxley in support of the classical reductionist program for biology. In spite of his constant criticism of ideal morphology, he was heavily influenced by aesthetic factors in his own theories. Ritterbush 1968, pp. 60–62, describes how Huxley's beliefs about the structure of protoplasm led him to postulate that slime dredged from the ocean was "a living substrate of naked jelly seemingly capable of generating simple marine organisms"—an *Urschleim*. The classification derived from the influence of the idea of organic form. The incident is still another support for the assertion that aesthetics and science are more than casually linked.

will be explored later. The essence of his position was an acceptance of strict mechanism in science but a rigid exclusion of a metaphysical materialism. His compromise was to oppose method to metaphysics and insist upon the relevance of mechanism to science and teleology to philosophy. The unsatisfactory nature of the resolution is obvious. As has been noted in the analysis of his early papers, he was already *scientifically* unhappy with all the implications of the machine analogy when it dealt with hierarchical levels and field phenomena. However, he had not yet articulated the full organismic paradigm that could carry him beyond the contradictions.

The next paragraphs of the introduction concentrated on a description of the neo vitalists and organicists whom he rejected. The principal sin attributed to such men as Russell, Haldane, and Driesch was the use of psychic categories of explanation—toying with Aristotelian finalism.[7] Needham then praised Lawrence J. Henderson, author of *The Fitness of the Environment* (1917), for having emphasized the reciprocal fitness of organism and environment, thereby abolishing any need for a special teleology of the organism. From one aspect both organism and environment exhibit a "universal teleology," but finalism is useless on the level of scientific explanation. Needham drew Whitehead into support for this position. Everything is an organism, but the concept is methodologically useless for science by virtue of its universal applicability in philosophy. Organisms are everywhere, so "the difference between the living and the non-living becomes a quantitative one, expressible in degrees of organization" (1931, p. 29). Needham was to express the relevance of Whitehead quite differently when he was expounding the legitimacy of his own scientific organicism. To remove any lingering doubt about the attitude toward science that he was advocating, Needham concluded the section with the assertions that biology is complicated physics and that abstraction as the method and mechanism as the form of explanation are necessary partners. He even felt that mature science would abandon model and analogy, as Eddington said physics did with the principle of indeterminacy. That his own neomechanism rested heavily on a metaphor was irrelevant to Needham's scientific faith of 1928.

Without ever abandoning a strict insistence on mathematical rigor, Needham was hardly a mechanist by the end of the third volume. Most

7. See chapter 1 above, pp. 18–20 and pp. 22–23 for a detailed exposition of Needham's position here.

of the epilegomena treated topics peripherally relevant to construction of an organismic paradigm. But under the subheading "Biochemistry and morphogenesis," discussion turned to Spemann and the organizer. Needham considered work on the nature of the organizer centrally important to biology. "If it turns out to be, as seems very likely, something partaking of the nature of a hormone, an extremely significant bridge will have been thrown across the ancient gulf between physico-chemical processes and their morphological manifestations" (1931, p. 1626). He speculated that the organizer was connected with Child's physiological gradients. From that point it was a short step to field theories. It is necessary to remember that Harrison thought Child's gradient explanations unhelpful because they were ambiguous about structure and form.[8] Needham, on the other hand, was much more tolerant of Child's theories, which lay behind much of his own later work on metabolic characteristics of the organizer region. In this sense Harrison was more purely organismic, or structuralist, than Needham. However, Needham interpreted Child's ideas of dominance of a region in organismic terms, insisting that physiological activity was not separable from structure. The concentration on a search for hormone-like molecules and on metabolic characteristics of the organizer region ensured that Needham's field was a material one befitting a biochemist. Hardly surprisingly, he never entertained an idea of true action at a distance, focusing instead on position effects and complex interactions of molecular systems.

Toward the end of the epilegomena Needham presented a list of thirty-two provisional generalizations for chemical embryology. Two will be touched on here in order to illustrate the extent to which by 1931 he was thinking beyond his earlier neomechanism. "Determination or chemodifferentiation takes place with reference to the whole organism; what any given part will develop into depends upon its position with reference to the whole" (1931, p. 1651). Driesch's generalization was referred by Needham not to any entelechy but to the notion of internal relationship, an idea borrowed from Joseph Woodger. Properties of parts were determined by the sorts of relationships maintained with neighboring parts within the whole. This

8. Professor G. Evelyn Hutchinson of Yale recalls discussing Child with Harrison in the 1930s. Harrison's chief objection seemed to be the lack of good *direct* evidence for metabolic gradients. He nonetheless had a student of Child, J. W. Buchanan, appointed so Osborn would have an axial gradient man (personal correspondence, July 4, 1971).

general rule translated into principles such as : "The cells of a developing embryo are internally related to each other in the sense that the
rate and plane of division of a given cell depend on its relations to the
neighboring cells and hence on its position in the whole" (p. 1651
[quoted from Woodger]). Other generalizations in the list emphasized
increase in complexity during development, establishment of gradient
systems and symmetrical plans, and regulation of form within boundary
conditions.

The section called "The organization of development and the
development of organization" contained two points of importance.
The first concerned the relation of biology to physics. Traditional
physics was incapable of explaining the development of form or
organized growth. Needham stressed that a new physics and chemistry
would be required. "But their present condition is not a stationary one
and much may be expected when the new concepts of physics, having
penetrated the realm of chemistry [see Langmuir] come at last to that
of embryology" (1931, p. 1659). The reference to Langmuir high-
lighted the nature of the expected change in physics and chemistry:
they would become sciences of structure and form, that is, they
themselves would operate from organismic perspectives. The second
critical point concerned the usefulness of the crystal analogy in biology.
Needham used crystals to emphasize intermediate organization and
levels. Form, or organization, appropriate to a level was immanent:
there was no controlling principle operating from without. Needham
used the term *Gestaltprinzip*, adopted from Ludwig von Bertalanffy, an
early Austrian advocate of organicism (later general systems theory).
The *Gestaltprinzip* preserved the grain of truth from theories of emergence that had been prominent in theoretical biology. The high degree
of organization in living systems had to be a consequence of fundamental properties of matter, but it had to be understood in terms of
organizing relations above the molecular level. Again Needham was
drawing from his friend Woodger. The legitimate autonomy of
biology lay in the expression of laws of integration proper to a particular
level. The unity of science derived from explicating connections
between levels not from abolition of the specific qualities of organized
systems.

In the developing embryo, then, we have a process more or less
analogous to the crystallizing solution, but one which reaches

much further up into the realm of organization. To say this is to state a problem, not to solve one, and just as physics and chemistry have in the past dealt with crystal-form and incorporated it into their world picture, so biology must do for animal form.[9]

Before following Needham into his first experiments on the chemical nature of the organizer, it is necessary to review the well-known history of the discovery of the extraordinary material in Hans Spemann's laboratory. Spemann had been working since the early years of this century on the problem of dependent versus self-differentiation, a direct outgrowth of seeds sown by Roux, founder of the science of developmental mechanics. In 1924 Hilde Mangold, working with Spemann on such a series of experiments, transplanted a piece of the dorsal lip of the blastopore of the newt *Triton cristatus* so that it was in contact with indifferent (undetermined) ectoderm of an early gastrula of *Triton taeniatus*. The operation resulted in the formation of a complete secondary axis; two embryos formed instead of one. The induced structures from the host were "organized" by the implanted material into a coherent whole. Spemann called the peculiar dorsal lip area of the embryo the organization-center.

Needham judged that "the nature of the organizer influence was from the first recognized to set a problem the solution of which would profoundly affect our picture of the process of development. It meant nothing less than the discovery of the relational factor in development."[10] One of the first speculations, put forth by Julian Huxley and then by C. M. Child, on the true nature of the organizer ascribed it to a Childian gradient of high metabolic activity. Needham felt that there was a lack of evidence for such an assertion and that in addition a much more pleasing hypothesis was that the organizer was a single chemical substance operating much like a hormone on target tissue. This hypothesis had the agreeable side benefit of furthering the union of Cambridge biochemistry and German Entwicklungsmechanik. The likelihood of a simple chemical solution for the organizer was enhanced by Spemann's 1931 discovery that material from the center would still induce after its cells were killed by crushing. That is, the

9. 1931, p. 1662. It would not be strictly accurate to maintain that Needham introduced the study of chemical embryology. One must reach at least to Herbst and his work on the effects of lithium ions on sea urchin development.

10. 1936, p. 84. All quotes from this work will be taken from the 1968 MIT Press paperback reprint.

organization center itself did not have to be organized to exhibit its remarkable effects. In 1932, four workers, including Holtfreter in Berlin-Dahlem, showed that the organizer influence was not abolished by boiling, thereby eliminating the action of an enzyme.

Holtfreter completely blew the top off the situation by demonstrating, also in 1932, that parts of the body not usually possessing inductor activity could acquire it from boiling or treatment with protein-denaturing agents such as alcohol or acetone. Later to cause considerable experimental and theoretical trouble was the fact that the very material on which organization capacity was tested, the ventral ectoderm of amphibians, was itself shown after boiling to be capable of inducing formation of a secondary embryonic axis. Eventually it was shown that the "organizer-hormone" was present in most adult tissues of the newt, and indeed, throughout the animal kingdom. Holtfreter obtained neural inductions in the newt using material from chick primitive streak while another worker achieved similar results with human cancer cells.[11] Holtfreter had developed an ingenious test system in addition to the *Einsteckung* method (implantation of test material into the blastocoele cavity), which O. Mangold discovered shortly after the original finding of the organizer. The Dahlem biologist cultivated parts of the embryo separately in dilute Ringer's solution with a bicarbonate buffer. He surrounded a piece of test material with two flaps of presumptive epidermis. By these methods he was able to obtain good induction of neural structures. But for Needham the most relevant results of Holtfreter and others up to 1933 were those that favored the hypothesis of a simple chemical organizer.

Both Needham and Waddington had been in Germany in 1933. That year sparked a fruitful collaboration lasting until Waddington left

11. Holtfreter, brilliant and persistent in his efforts, seems to have been something of a thorn in the side of the Freiberg body of hopes for the organization center. Spemann was likely to favor slightly vitalistic explanations for the nature of his discovery; a simple chemical, least of all one of confusing specificity, was not an attractive candidate. He seems to have been less than cordial toward Holtfreter, with whom Waddington, a major collaborator with Needham and an important link with German biology, worked for a time in 1933. Waddington visited the laboratory of O. Mangold in Berlin in 1932 in order to learn techniques of amphibian operations. The British embryologist reported in a conversation on March 3, 1971, that Spemann was not interested in cooperating with his research goals at the time. Waddington had published a short paper on the chick organizer in 1930, after he had gone to the Strangeways Laboratory around 1928 in order to work on such problems. He had switched his concentration from fossils to embryos in order to satisfy more readily his interest in genetics. He then focused on the organizer simply because it was the most exciting problem in the embryology of the period.

Cambridge in 1939 for Edinburgh and more concentration on genetics. Before starting experiments on the organizer, both men were firmly grounded in organismic perspectives, and this fact was to affect their interpretations of laboratory results. Needham's work in this second experimental phase will be examined in four parts: a look at three papers from 1934 to 1936 on the physicochemical nature of the organizer, a series of investigations with E. J. Boell on metabolic characteristics relating to the liberation of the organizer, a 1937 paper on the chemical aspects of fields, and finally study with collaborators on the action mechanism of the organizer hormone, especially in relation to effects on fibrous proteins.

Needham's first paper on the organizer came when he was already hot on the trail of the anticipated chemical solution (Nedham, Waddington, and Needham 1934). It was known, for instance, that the suspected substance was resistant to boiling and to freezing and was not extracted from tissue by alcohol. Furthermore, if a piece of non-inducing ectoderm (presumptive epidermis) were implanted into the dorsal lip of the blastopore and allowed to pass inward into the roof of the archenteron, it acquired inductor power equivalent to that of the normal organization center. Such a fact was difficult to explain by a metabolic gradient theory but lent itself readily to some kind of diffusion process. Also, Holtfreter showed that pieces of tissue from blastulas or young gastrulas taken from regions distant from the organization center would undergo considerable differentiation when they were implanted into the peritoneal cavity of older larvae. On the other hand, similar pieces of tissue cultured *in vitro* underwent no neural differentiation. Something from *in vivo* conditions was acting on the donor tissue. It was likely the normal inducing agent acting by way of the peritoneal fluid. Other examples of inductions taking place through a liquid medium (Wolffian lens regeneration) were known and argued strongly for a hormone-like action.

The Needhams' and Waddington's publication reported early experiments with true cell-free extracts of the organizer region. Neural inductions were obtained with the extract after cell debris was spun out by centrifugation.

> The embryos were then ground up with anhydrous sodium sulphate, to absorb all water, and thoroughly extracted with solvents such as ether and petrol-ether. Again activity was found

in the extract, strongly indicating that the organizer-hormone, for such it could now legitimately be called, was of a fatty, lipoidal, or sterolic character, and so soluble in organic solvents.[12]

After describing the experiments, a distinction at the crux of the organicist view of the organizer was made. To attribute all the effects of the organization center to a single chemical substance would have been a classical reductionist explanation. But the postulate of a morphogenetic hormone was integrated with field thinking, so that the resulting form of explanation was a model of Needham's goal of bridging chemistry and morphogenesis.

Induction was considered to be the result of the interaction of three systems: the graft, the overlying host ectoderm, and the host organization center. The host ectoderm had to be competent to respond to the morphogenetic stimulus. At least two processes, or aspects of the same complex process, were seen to be involved in the determination of the host ectoderm to participate in the formation of a secondary embryonic axis. The first process was the "determination of the character of that axis." A number of experiments had revealed that the grafted tissue often influenced the regional character of the result. The basis of this specificity seemed to involve a set of complex interactions of a field nature. Determination of the presence of an axis was called evocation, whereas determination of its regional nature was called individuation. "In the ordinary induction, one of these determinations, evocation, is always performed by the graft, while the other, individuation, is performed by the graft and the host working together, either in a cooperative or an antagonistic manner" (Needham, Waddington, and Needham 1934, pp. 408, 409).

The authors reasoned that evocation was the result of a simple chemical stimulus, and they called their postulated morphogenetic hormone the evocator. The more interesting problem was individuation, a process that Needham felt could not be elicited by dead organizers or organizer extracts. Nevertheless, the 1934 paper dealt with efforts to identify the evocator not to unravel the knot of individuation phenomena. In fact, Needham, in contrast to Waddington's later concern for chreods, was never to probe the process experimentally, although he was to participate in further theoretical elaboration around the concept.

12. 1936, p. 86. The Einsteckung technique was used in these experiments.

Focusing on the evocator, Needham judged that the experiments strongly hinted at a lipoidal, likely steroid, nature. Although only weak neural inductions had been produced with the ether extracts, a relatively sophisticated statistical treatment of data justified the opinion that the reactions obtained were significant and that the difficulty to be resolved in the future was technical—better purification of the active substance. A large series of control experiments resulted in no neural inductions at all. Since it had been amply demonstrated that the evocator could be liberated from normally inactive tissue, the suggestion that the substance existed in a bound form was obvious. Only in cells ordinarily involved in inductions would active material be free. Such a hypothesis was pregnant with experimental expectations, and study of the processes involved in release of the evocator occupied much of Needham's time. In this light the results of Fischer and Wehmeier that glycogen derived from adult newt liver was active could be assimilated into the Cambridge workers' perspective. It was later (1935) demonstrated that the glycogen was indeed contaminated by an ether-soluble substance; pure glycogen was inactive. The possible involvement of glycogen in the normal masking of the evocator in the dorsal blastopore lip stimulated Needham to study the metabolism of that region in later work.[13]

The opinion that the evocator was sterol-like in nature was based on three main pieces of biochemical evidence: the active material was ether soluble, was present in the unsaponifiable fraction of the ether-soluble extract, and was precipitable with digitonin. These suggestive results were followed up by several additional experiments that tended to confirm the hypothesis. In 1936 Needham published two papers with a number of collaborators; the first examined activation of the evocator and the second expanded the evidence pointing to its steroid

13. It should be made clear that the biochemistry of the 1930s was technically unable to unravel the issues Needham, Waddington, and others were facing. The 1966 paper on the isolation of the lac repressor in bacteria by Gilbert and Miller-Hill highlights the immense difference in the technical capacity of biochemistry applied to superficially similar problems in 1966 compared to 1934. But more than technical problems derailed the train heading for a chemical solution of Spemann's organizer phenomena (see Goodfield 1969). The Cambridge scientists had high hopes for the purification of a simple evocator partly because they conceptually separated evocation as a process from the more complex individuation. When, by the mid- to late 1930s it had become clear that inductions could be obtained with virtually anything, including methylene blue and a wide variety of artificial substances, the legitimacy of such a theoretical distinction was less obvious but still defensible. However, these remarks take us ahead of the story as it unfolded.

character. In the later paper (Waddington et al. 1936) the authors confirmed the presence of an evocator substance in the digitonin precipitate of the unsaponifiable material of ether extracts of crude glycogen. In addition they began the fractionation of sterol portions of the unsaponifiable material derived from adult pig liver. They hoped that fractionation would narrow the field of choice for the natural active evocator. Finally this paper weighed against an alternative suggestion that the nonsteroid lipid kephalin was an active evocator by demonstrating that acetone extracts of brain, which should not contain kephalin, were active and that kephalin preparations were still active after destruction of the lipid by saponification. Thus, they reasoned, kephalin fractions had been active due to contamination with a steroid. Linking the evocator with the sterols was made almost irresistible by the attraction of contemporary work on steroid hormones and carcinogenic compounds. There was little doubt that this class of chemicals had immense biological significance; a steroid morphogenetic hormone would be a pleasing result.

In the first 1936 paper (Waddington, Needham, and Brachet 1936) the collaborators attempted to integrate their opinions about the chemical nature of the evocator with a probe of the mechanism of its activation. Needham was trying to unify his perspective with Child's and Huxley's. Huxley had compared the organizer experiments to isolation of portions of the axial gradient system of lower organisms (e.g., coelenterates); an isolated part of such systems was said to reconstitute a dominant region. Establishment of a secondary organization center in amphibians was compared with the dominant region of an axial gradient. Although an axial gradient could not be directly active in performing inductions, it could act through the liberation of active substances in privileged regions of the gradient system. Child had always favored a gradient of metabolic rate, particularly respiratory rate. Accordingly, Needham et al. attempted to raise the metabolic rate of isolated fragments of ectoderm and then test treated implants for neural induction capacity. The results with methylene blue, a vital dye that acts as a respiratory catalyst, were positive. Obviously, methylene blue bears no resemblance to any natural evocator. Either the trail seeming to lead to the purification of a natural sterol-like inductor was a false one, or else the dye acted by liberating the natural substance.

These speculations developed into a tentative theory of the evocator.

Several substances that were active inductors are the following: ether extracts of crude liver glycogen; the unsaponifiable digitonin-pre-cipitable fraction of adult liver; certain synthetic estrogenic hydro-carbons; thymonucleic acid, muscle adenylic acid, oleic, linolenic, and other higher fatty acids; crude kephalin; and finally methylene blue. In addition several processes applied to gastrula ectoderm caused that tissue to beome capable of inducing neural structures from a second piece of ectoderm. The processes included normal invagination through the blastopore, treatment with organic solvents, freezing, boiling, crushing, drying, and finally treatment with methylene blue. The interpretation of all these data rested on a continuing assumption that evocation must be specific, that is, performed in eggs of the same species by the same substance. Decision between sterols and acids was made on the basis of dosage required. Sterols would induce neural differentiation in very low concentrations similar to those of natural active hormones. Acids induced only if present in large amounts. Other treatments were postulated to act by liberating the natural evocator. Perhaps also, the evocator was contained as an impurity (e.g., as with kephalin). The overwhelming difficulty of this line of reasoning was the impossibility of deciding whether the implant acting as a successful stimulus for induction contained the natural inductor or only unmasked it in the test system (indirect induction). This situation posed both a theoretical and a practical road block that was not effectively removed by work on induction and the evocator in the 1930s. But remaining to tempt the biochemist in Needham's soul was the range of specific, repeatable inductions subsumed under the theory of the organizer.

The association of a sterol-like evocator with glycogen was next explored. It was known that as invagination proceeded through the blastopore lips, glycogen disappeared from the cells. The obvious course was to study how glycogen loss during invagination linked up with overall glycogen metabolism during development. Brachet and Needham attempted to probe this problem in 1935 by estimating total glycogen in the egg and also glycogen bound with protein. The data were inconclusive, but the suspicion that the evocator existed in a bound glycogen–protein complex was strengthened. Any treatment denaturing the protein, such as boiling or exposure to organic solvent, would liberate the evocator.

A more detailed effort to study the evocator and glycogen metabolism was made in a series of papers published with E. J. Boell in 1939.[14] Boell, in Cambridge on a Rockefeller fellowship, was an excellent technical manipulator, and the experiments were conducted on microgram quantities of embryonic material. The measurements were the finest made up to that time. The Cartesian diver, a device first described in 1648 by a student of Galileo, Raffaele Magiotti, was essentially an ultramicromanometer 1,500 times more sensitive than the standard Warburg manometer. The first paper established that the dorsal blastopore lip (i.e., the organization center of the amphibian gastrula) "has a higher anaerobic glycolysis and a higher ammonia production than the ventral ectoderm. The difference, established by statistical test, is of the order of three times" (Boell, Needham, and Rogers 1939, p. 354).

The next step was the effort to abolish the difference in anaerobic metabolism. The ultimate aim was to show that the alteration in this particular component of metabolism was related to releasing the masked evocator from ventral ectoderm. Dinitro-o-cresol, a dye believed to act upon mechanisms of carbohydrate utilization, raised the metabolic level of the ventral ectoderm more than it raised the rate of the dorsal lip region; that is, the lower metabolic rate was preferentially stimulated. A similar phenomenon had been observed by Boell in grasshopper embryos in diapause, although the observed increase in respiratory activity in the orthopterans was probably due to protein, not carbohydrate, breakdown. Analogies to sea urchin eggs also existed, and the authors thought there was reason to believe that the observed effect of the nitrophenol was relevant to normal respiration. "In general we may say that wide variations in metabolic activity exist in correlation with various physiological and morphogenetic states. The regions of high activity may or may not be in a condition of maximum possible activity, but the regions or states of low activity are certainly damped down" (Boell and Needham 1939a, p. 361). The authors felt it was significant that the evocator was normally liberated in a region of high metabolic activity. However, the crucial second step, demonstrating that dinitro-o-cresol brought about a liberation of the evocator in pieces of ventral ectoderm, was not successful. The observed effect on glycolysis remained ambiguous.

14. E. J. Boell, Joseph Needham, and Veronica Rogers 1939; E. J. Boell and Joseph Needham 1939a, 1939b; E. J. Boell, Henri Koch, and Joseph Needham 1939.

Attention was then turned to oxygen consumption of regions of the young *Amblystoma* embryos. The Cartesian diver apparatus was modified for these measurements to allow a level of precision comparable to the above tests. The level of O_2 use of the dorsal lip region and the ventral ectoderm did not differ significantly. When the respiratory quotient was examined (ratio of oxygen consumption to carbon dioxide evolution), it was found that the "dorsal lip region shows a greater trend towards unity than does the ventral ectoderm." But the respiratory quotient was not constant during the period examined. "We have to do, therefore, with a progressive alteration of the quality of metabolism during gastrulation, and not with its quantity" (Boell, Koch, and Needham 1939, p. 386). These interesting results made possible by ingenious use of the diver remained ambiguous in relation to the postulated evocator complex.

Needham did not solve the problem of the evocator before events led him into China and the history of science, and after the war other workers on the organizer approached inductors from much modified viewpoints. Nonetheless, it is relevant to follow the Cambridge biochemist in his opinions on the relationship of the postualated evocator to field problems and to go with him through his last set of experimental manipulations. For it is here, where his organicist framework is most clear, that he converged with Harrison and Weiss.

The hypothesis of a sterol-like morphogenetic hormone appealed to Needham for reasons beyond the implication of that class of molecules for important responses in many biological systems. Molecules related to cholesterol formed liquid crystals with intriguing properties. The structure of steroids was only coming to be understood around 1930. Needham speculated that the paracrystalline structures oriented protein molecules in the neighborhood. The orienting effect could be transmitted throughout a region, triggering a transformation in the field parameters of the system. The concept of a hormone was enlarged by including the notion of a molecule that propagated its effects by contact without traveling to all target points. "We are left, then, with the conception of a sterol-like substance being liberated at a given point in the developing system and 'radiating' its organising power from that spot" (1936, p. 95). Part of the specificity of the reaction would depend on the proteins in the reacting system; for example, the morphogenetic hormone would trigger the proteins in the flat neural plate to reorient themselves in such a way as to result in the formation of a tube. The focus on structure and orientation in the reacting system was invoked by Harrison in his consideration of amphibian limb formation.

In a paper published in 1937 Needham considered the chemical aspects of morphogenetic fields (pp. 66–81). The heart of the paper was "its suggestion that, although the chemical aspects of morphogenetic fields are exceedingly difficult to grasp, nevertheless the new understanding of proteins as crystalline fibers capable of being oriented in certain definite patterns by active substances or hormones may go some way to helping our imagination" (p. 78). The contemporary work on proteins encouraged Needham to think in terms of a "subtle intra- and inter-cellular lattice, carrying the properties of polarity and symmetry, and capable of far-reaching temporary disarrangement, without loss of integration." The evocator, and indeed the whole hierarchy of inductors, would stimulate irreversible distortions and re-orientations of molecular systems. Finally, "the new and ever more stable equilibria into which the whole molecular assemblage falls under the influence of these substances are not isolated, but are related to each other according to laws which present the appearance of field laws" (p. 79). All the essential components of an organismic field theory are clearly present in these ideas. The similarity to Harrison's general theory of development is striking.

Needham believed that fields were distinguished from simple geographic regions of the embryo by three criteria: any given point within the field force had to possess a given quality, a given direction, and a given intensity. Fields were judged in terms of instability and successive equilibrium positions. Waddington reasoned that "a field is a system of order such that the position taken up by unstable entities in one portion of the system bears a definite relation to the position taken up by unstable entities in other portions." Behavior of cells was, within certain boundaries, a function of position within the whole. Many of the organizational forces of fields were "to some extent on a suprachemical level" (p. 71). Needham saw the work of D'Arcy Thompson as a significant but chemically unspecified root of legitimate field thinking. Needham hoped that his work on the evocator, coupled with a sophisticated understanding of proteins and paracrystalline structures, would give a firm biochemical content to morphogenetic fields. One goal was to account for the multiplicity of biological fields in contrast to the relatively few kinds of physical fields.

Needham fully realized that field theory occupied a peculiar position within biology and that the concept often carried an immense weight of "thought experiments." Nonetheless, he held that field thinking was a "powerful aid to the codification of *Gestaltungsgesetze*, the rules of morphogenetic order."[15] Needham rejected the geometrical fields of Gurwitsch and drew from the speculation of Weiss and Waddington. The basic notion was, in Waddington's words, that of "wholes organizing themselves" (Needham 1936, p. 102). Fields invited the introduction of topographical models and reasoning. For example, Needham described, a kind of qualitative mathematical model of an amphibian neurula.

> If the whole of one side of an amphibian neurula is mapped in hemispherical projection, the probabilities of organ-formation can be represented by a landscape of hills, the contour-lines being the "isobars," as it were, of probability ... it would be tempting to make a parallel between these concentric zones of organ probability and the concentric zones of increasing randomness (probability of molecular orientation) which later on we shall consider as surrounding a central polarising molecule or paracrystalline molecular aggregate. [pp. 106–07]

In sum, Needham saw field law as a dynamic description of the establishment of order and form during development. He was convinced that fields were an advance over static anatomical description in embryology. Fields provided a rich source of images for the experimental task of concretization.

In this context Needham in his last experiments switched emphasis from the characterization of the evocator to the second term of the organizer problem, the individuation field. The work was analogous to the investigations that Harrison undertook with Astbury in 1939–40, that is, a search for oriented protein molecules in a field system. The underlying conviction was that protein shape changes could throw light upon gross morphological transformations. Accordingly, Needham joined with A. S. C. Lawrence and Shih-Chang Shen in "Studies on the anomalous viscosity and flow-birefringence of protein solutions" (Lawrence, Needham, and Shen 1944). Neurulation was the focus of

---

15. 1936, p. 99. The German word derived from Ludwig von Bertalanffy, the organicist introduced to Needham by Woodger.

attention. Could observed changes in cell shape (elongation) be related to increase in size, number, or axial ratio of anisometric protein particles? The technique employed was a special viscometer. Elongated (anisometric) molecules reacted differently to shear than spherical ones; the difference was referred to as anomalous viscosity. Protein solutions prepared from pieces of neural tube and from regions on the embryo unlikely to possess special fiber properties were compared in their reactions to shear forces and in their optical properties under the experimental conditions (flow birefringence). The basic result showed that "in the amphibian embryo there is a protein or group of proteins in the total euglobulin class which spreads instantaneously into a surface film having the property of anomalous flow. Its molecules must therefore pass readily into the fibrillar state."[16]

In the companion paper to the first, the authors joined with Margaret Miall in studying flow birefringence and anomalous viscosity of three groups of proteins and in speculating on the biological significance of the results. The group A molecules, myosin and tobacco mosaic virus nucleoprotein, were clearly elongated before denaturation treatments. They showed flow anomaly and birefringence in bulk phase, and their role in fiber formation was obvious. Group B, which included the proteins from amphibian neurulas, showed anomalous viscosity and birefringence only in surface films, not in bulk. The interpretation was that such molecules will form fibrillar structures after surface denaturation, an effect with possible *in vivo* significance. A third group, C, showed flow anomaly neither in bulk nor in surface film. These molecules, including insulin and amphibian egg jelly, were thought to be spherical.

Throughout this work the importance of fibers to Needham's concept of biological organization is evident. In the experiments the authors were concerned with four aspects of postulated biological significance:

16. Lawrence, Needham, and Shen 1944, p. 231. The species were *Rana temporaria* and *Bufo vulgaris*. In 1942 Needham most clearly related the notion of anomalous flow to structured protoplasm. "Protoplasm undoubtedly shows anomalous viscosity. Pfeiffer and others have found that the velocity of its forced shearing flow, as in a capillary tube, increases with increasing force at first slowly, later more quickly. For Newtonian liquids the relation, however, is linear. Also protoplasm has a 'yield value,' *i.e.*, requires a specially large initial force to start the flow (cf. thixotrophy). The viscosity of true liquids is unaffected by pressure, but that of protoplasm greatly decreases as the pressure increases. The anomalous flow of protoplasm is paralleled by many non-living colloids . . . if they consist of anisometric particles which mechanically interfere with each other's motion" (1942, p. 661).

1. the location of protein fractions showing elongated particle shape, and the participation of these in the architecture of living cells ... ;

2. the mutual interactions of substrates and enzymes, when the latter are themselves elongated particles, involving changes, reversible or irreversible, in the configuration of the enzyme micells;

3. the formation of elongated molecules and micelles by living cells—the processes by which they are "spun";

4. the formation of microscopically visible fibers, as *e.g.*, in connective tissue. [1944, p. 203]

The use of the fiber and tissue metaphor amply expresses Needham's mature conception of the resolution of the field–particle dichotomy in biological field theory. It remains now to trace the biochemist's philosophical development as it paralleled and enriched his experimental perspective.

Until the founding of the Theoretical Biology Club, Needham was intrigued by the mechanism–vitalism controversy and formulated his own preference within the confines of its underlying paradigm. An essay composed in 1925 highlights his preoccupations (1925), while the first article in a collection of essays that appeared in 1930 extends the position reached in those early years (1930*b*, pp. 15–43). The fundamental tenet of his neomechanism was the belief that physicochemical explanation must be extended to cover all natural phenomena. The mechanistic program alone had resulted in progress in scientific knowledge; vitalism had always been obscurantist. Nonetheless, there was an important truth in vitalism: concern for the element of consciousness, the inner lining of the world. Thus Needham found himself forced to accept a radical dualism. Mechanism was necessary to science but could never deal with consciousness. Its success might be due only to the peculiar construction of our minds and have nothing to say about the structure of the natural world. He rejected any split between organic and inorganic but preserved the division between mind and body. He did not envision mind and body as ultimate categories but as aspects of reality that must not be confused.

Needham reserved the name *scientific naturalism* for the philosophy, best expressed by Jacques Loeb, that scientific method was the sole legitimate approach to experience. The appeal of Loeb's position to a biologist was immense, but it had to be rejected nevertheless. Vitalism's alternative, however, ruled out the possibility of science. From the beginning Needham maintained that "the concept of organization is definitely not an affair of the reflective judgment, but a very legitimate field for scientific experiment and calculation" (1928*b*, p. 80). In later writings Needham preserved his insistence on rigorous analysis. But "The sceptical biologist" contained a revealing treatment of the legitimacy of analogy and metaphor, a treatment appropriate to Needham the neomechanist but discarded by the mature organicist. Ideal science formed "a closed circle of conceptions, each depending on the others for its meaning. . . . No gap can be found anywhere in the cycle . . . and this mechanistic scheme of the inorganic is a very great part of the achievement of science" (1930*b*, p. 22). Still borrowing from Eddington, Needham insisted that the path to such a self-sufficient system consisted of measurement and the ruthless weeding out of anthropomorphic images. Such images were cracks for final causes to seep through. Ideally, mature science would do entirely without analogy and concrete models.

Because Needham withheld metaphysical validity from the mechanical world view, he asserted "its universality but [denied] its finality" (p. 29). That formulation led him to see science as pure tactic, "only methodologically representing truth." The attitude of science was essential, but only for subjective reasons. Neither the mechanical nor the finalistic views had any real counterparts in nature. Science simply proceeded *as if* its description of nature were true. So in summary, Needham regarded "the mechanistic view of the world as a legitimate methodological distortion, capable of application to any phenomenon whatever, and possessing no value at all as a metaphysical doctrine. Such a standpoint let us call Neo-mechanism" (p. 33). Needham had some expectations of a unified perspective on the world and hoped for a welding of the metaphysical and mechanistic visions by the operation of "intuition." The typical antirationalism of positivist science is evident here. This position was radically subjectivist and was emphatically discarded under the impact of two influences: Marxism and the organicism of J. H. Woodger.

The article entitled "Biology as a field of contest between Aristotle and Plato" shows the first influence of Woodger and represents a transition position for Needham (1932, pp. 99–125). The paper began with a description of the debt of science to the Plato of the *Timaeus*, to whom we owe our appreciation of mathematics and general laws. But throughout its history biology was founded on the classificatory insights of Aristotle, a morphologist and a systematist. To the first great biologist we owe especially the distinction between form and matter. But to him the tendency toward vitalism has also been ascribed. The unification of Plato and Aristotle in a full science was one of Needham's hopes.

Needham associated Plato with the development of theoretical biology, which until 1930 had been concerned only with the mechanics of evolution and speculation about the nature and origin of life. It had been none too rigorous or logical in its methods and often issued in uncritical vitalism, but Needham believed the need for it was great. "Yet it is extremely important to realize that we need theoretical biology at least as much as the more practical studies of experimental workers, and until we get it the structure of biology will remain ... a medley of unorganized *ad hoc* hypotheses."[17] Furthermore, the Cambridge biochemist now explicitly rejected contemporary physics and chemistry as the key to biology: "It may be very well that such questions as the mechanism of differentiation and determination in the developing egg are completely insoluble as long as we try to reduce the phenomena to terms capable of fusion with the classical physics and the classical chemistry" (1932, p. 107). New developments in logical theory were particularly promising for the progress of biology. There were rigorous methods of analysis, such as topography, that were pregnant for the embryologist prepared to go beyond the confines of static anatomy or of simplistic dynamic explanations such as Loeb's tropisms.

The central problem of the new theoretical biology was organization. Aristotle's form term was transformed into organization, and his matter was conceived as energy in the new framework. Needham presented an extended discussion of the analogy of crystal and organism, a discussion relying on an organicist understanding of analogy and the significance of hierarchy. He drew from Bertalanffy's *Kritische Theorie der Formbildung* (1933). The historical development of organisms had constituted "a real flowering of organizing relations, about which there

---

17. 1932, p. 107. The belief expressed here was formulated in light of Woodger's article in *Mind* (1930b).

was nothing miraculous, for what we used to call matter was only waiting to produce them when given the opportunity."[18] The organizing principle of Bertalanffy was called *Gestaltprinzip* or *Ganzheit-factor*. It differed essentially from Driesch's Aristotelian entelechy because it was totally immanent in matter and could be studied by analytical science, albeit a science widened in its self-conception. "Organic coordination appears where it was absent before, but not as something fundamentally mysterious and anomic, something which must be taken as a postulate and not further explained."[19]

Organization was the principal problem at all levels of integration.

> When we consider the fact that the protoplasm of the living cell is undoubtedly polyphasic, containing as it were, globules within globules, each separate kind with its own organization and potentialities which it cannot overpass, we are able to visualize the immense complexity which the simplest unit of life must have within it. [1932, pp. 114–15]

Facing the facts of organization was equivalent to moving toward the union of morphology and biophysics. Perhaps here was the beginning of biology, not its completion. Organization was measurable but only for an expanded mathematics. In any case it was certain that the concept of chaotic, homogeneous matter had to be replaced by measurable, structured systems of energy, and static form gave way to internal organizing relations. "The hierarchy of relationships, from the molecular structure of carbon compounds at one end to the equilibrium between species in ecological wholes at the other, will probably be the guiding concept in biology henceforth" (p. 117). The

18. Needham 1932, p. 112. Included in the notion of organizing relations was determination of developmental fate by position within the whole. The "pre-relativity" understanding of position had given way to Woodger's and Whitehead's notion that spatial relations are internal organizing relations. The result was "a new range of theoretical possibilities capable of being expressed in accurate mathematical terms, and capable of fusion with the physics of space-time" (pp. 121–22).

19. Ibid., pp. 112–13. Needham distinguished two kinds of theoretical biology: that associated with J. S. Haldane and E. S. Russell and that of Bertalanffy and Woodger. Needham felt that the former passively acquiesced to organized wholes. The latter knew there was much to learn from the crystallographer and the mathematical physicist. Needham came to appreciate Bertalanffy through the urgings of Woodger. In a letter to Woodger dated November 12, 1929, Needham said he believed that his difficulties with the Austrian were purely verbal and would be overcome quickly. He said that he could never feel similarly about E. S. Russell. Needham and Bertalanffy carried on an extensive correspondence from 1929 to 1946, interrupted by the war.

organicist, or structuralist, building blocks of boundaries or limits and a scale of integration are definitely operative for Needham.

The organismic paradigm was strengthened and explicated in the context of a most interesting paradigm community, the Theoretical Biology Club. The founding of the club was preceded by a fruitful exchange between Needham and Woodger. Needham met J. H. Woodger in November 1929, when the author of *Biological Principles* spoke at Cambridge.[20] Woodger had written Needham a long letter in May 1928 but never mailed it. The letter contained a detailed criticism of Needham's subjectivism. Woodger argued that it was impossible to refute the metaphysical pretensions of Driesch's vitalism when one's view of science was restricted to methodological claims. Woodger thought that Needham needed to enlarge his outlook on science, particularly by including in it "more of an organic perspective." Discussion about the content of such an organic view was extensive. In a letter dated February 26, 1929, Needham commented on the significance of molecular structure and formulated a definition of enzyme that was full of organismic biases.

> Is not the modern view of enzyme action very important for your position? The fact that nobody has ever isolated an enzyme as a chemical entity in a pure state has led biochemists to abandon the hope that anyone ever will, and by all the best people enzymes

20. Needham remarked in conversation in May 1970 that the publication of *Biological Principles* marked the end of the particular debate between neovitalists and mechanists precipitated by Driesch in the late nineteenth century. It is debatable whether many biologists read Woodger's tome, or were influenced by it if they did, but it did make a difference to Needham and Waddington. It appears that a critical passage in the book was the one in chapter 7 that stated that the "term 'vitalism' should be restricted to theories which postulate some entity in the living organism *in addition to* the chemical elements C, H, N, O, P, etc., plus organizing relations" (1936, p. 7).

The other publications of Woodger that had some impact for British organicists appeared in three parts in 1930 and 1931 as "The 'concept of organism' and the relation between embryology and genetics" (1930*a*, 1931). Woodger soon turned to a study of the axiomatic principles of the science of biology. Always impressed by symbolic logic and Russell's and Whitehead's monumental joint venture, Woodger gave himself entirely to the axiomatic method. This emphasis marked the end of his importance for Needham and Waddington and for organismic biology. Woodger's ultimate positions were radically nominalist. His more inclusive early organicism of *Biological Principles* was not buttressed by the socialist political and philosophical perspectives of Needham, Bernal, and Waddington—a fact that might shed some light on his later development. But Woodger's later extreme preoccupation with logical issues was rooted in a lifelong attention to maximum clarity of scientific and philosophical concepts. He became progressively more isolated in his work and tragically resulted in talking to no one.

are now regarded as sets of conditions (fields of force, residual valencies, etc.) associated with particular kinds of colloidal aggregates.

This astonishing attitude toward enzymes for a man about to enter upon a search for the simple chemical evocator is enlightening.[21]

Woodger wrote back on November 29, 1929, after his Cambridge lecture on science and religion, that he found Needham's remarks on molecular structure and pattern important. He added that he saw any biological "thing" as an organized entity (Whitehead). Properties of biological parts that change in isolation are then relational properties. Moreover, Woodger viewed metabolism as "the seat of perpetual rhythmical changes, with a varying rhythm to boot." He concluded by stressing that what was needed, and what Needham should address himself to, was a "logical epistemology of chemical theory."

In the spring of 1932 Needham, Waddington, and Woodger were together at Oxford and the conversation turned to the possibility of a "biotheoretical gathering" in the coming summer. Woodger wrote Needham on April 30, 1932, to suggest topics. The list included:

1. The bearing of modern work in logic on *Theorienbildung* in natural science.

2. The relation between chemical concepts and biological ones.

3. The relation between "descriptive" and "experimental" branches of biology.

4. The mutual relations of taxonomy, genetics, embryology, and phylogeny.

5. The analysis of current notions in embryology, "determination," "potency," "segregation," etc.

Needham wrote back (August 5, 1932) that he approved Woodger's ideas for the meeting at Tanhurst and that he preferred the second topic for discussion. He suggested three additional participants:

---

21. It was not known in those days that enzymes were proteins, and the exciting realm of molecular form determining function remained to be explored. Haldane, in a 1924 lecture defined an enzyme as "an organic catalyst of unknown composition," presumably unintentionally implying that when such a catalyst was fully characterized, it ceased to be an enzyme! (personal correspondence with G. E. Hutchinson, July 4, 1971).

L. L. Whyte, a mathematical physicist interested in biology; A. D. Ritchie, a Manchester physiologist; and J. D. Bernal, a Communist crystallographer who had worked on the structure of sterols.

The first meeting took place in mid-August. In commenting on the conference, Needham told Woodger that Waddington and Dorothy Wrinch had decided to work together in using topological models to measure differentiation rate and intensity.[22] Needham, "in harmony with my collectivist politics," favored a wider team than Wrinch and Waddington. He suggested, especially because Woodger had started them all thinking about topology in 1931, that everyone except Bernal and Dorothy Needham should join in the project. A second meeting took place in 1932, this time including also B. P. Weisner, a Viennese Jew living in Scotland and working on sex hormones. He had expressed to Needham an interest in the relevance of analysis situs (topology) to biology.

It would be instructive to look more carefully at the topics treated in the first meeting of the paradigm group to which Needham was to dedicate his *Order and Life*.[23] Using solid geometrical figures to illustrate his points, Waddington gave a paper on allelomorphic genes in *Drosophila* and another on the organizer, self-differention, and unstable equilibria in development. Needham and Waddington together talked about the idea of fields. Dorothy Wrinch discussed ways of assessing the complexity of morphological forms and then enlarged on "geometrical botany." J. D. Bernal developed his ideas on the junction of physics and chemistry and treated hierarchy and emergent evolution. He outlined a scale of form reaching from quantum mechanical systems to the metazoa. Bernal, calling for a "neo-cytology of proteins," noted the relevance of such work to field theory. However, Bernal's greatest contribution to the meetings of that year was probably his explanation of liquid crystals. It is obvious from studying Needham's notes from the meeting that many of his published remarks on paracrystals were drawn from Bernal's informal conversations.[24] Weisner tried to sketch his notion of a unit of order with nonatomistic constituents. Black

22. Participants also included Max Black, who later wrote the provocative books on analogy and metaphor in science that were cited in the chapter 1 above.

23. The Theoretical Biology Club continued to meet at least until 1936 and exchange continued until World War II.

24. The description of the TBC meetings comes from penciled notes kept in Needham's files. I am indebted to him for xerox copies of discussions held in 1932 and 1936.

talked on language error and regions of vagueness in concepts, illustrating his points with the idea of organism. Finally Woodger, the host, outlined his notions on collections and ordered systems and on maps and cones in analyzing genetic relations. This superficial list of the concerns of the TBC members should make it clear that the elements of nonvitalistic organicism, or structuralism in contemporary terminology, were precisely the bonds comenting the workers. The organismic paradigm involved the convergence of thought from mathematics, experimental embryology, biochemistry, biophysics, protein chemistry, logic, and language theory. By 1932 the paradigm was fully operative in Needham's thought; the former mechanistic paradigm no longer fostered the interesting questions.

Needham tried to construct an institute around the new paradigm commitments but was unable to obtain needed financing. Beginning in 1934 he corresponded with Dr. Tisdale of the Rockefeller Foundation, which was then interested in fostering study on the borderlines of traditional disciplines. In July Needham submitted a long memorandum outlining a plan for an Institute for Physico-chemical Morphology that would incorporate experimental embryology, descriptive morphology (later dropped from projections), tissue culture, chemical embryology, and theoretical embryology. Scientists at Cambridge would work closely with those at the Strangeways Laboratories who had long engaged in valuable embryological researches in Britain. Personnel suggested for the institute were, logically, Bernal for crystallography and chemistry, Wrinch for geometrical morphology, Honor Fell of Strangeways for tissue culture, Waddington for experimental embryology, and Needham for chemical embryology. Cambridge was experiencing a financial squeeze in the years before the war and was unable to grant its share of money for required building and salaries. Therefore, the Rockefeller Foundation withdrew after supporting a histologist for several years. By 1938 the idea was dead, but by that year work on the organizer itself had entered a crisis from which it did not recover. The reasons are controversial and complex, but the success of Needham's institute certainly would have altered the course of biological investigation in England after the 1930s. Instead, factors combined to break up the collaboration of members of the paradigm community, and World War II finally sealed the issue.[25]

25. Discussion of the institute is contained in notes and letters in Needham's files from 1934 to 1938. The first memorandum develops an interesting history of embryology and biochemistry in England from Needham's standpoint.

The second major influence that directed Needham to organismic thinking in his work was socialism.[26] In 1941 in an essay entitled "Metamorphoses of scepticism" he surveyed his personal intellectual history and evaluated the impact of Marxism (1943, pp. 7–28). He had divided up experience into mutually exclusive, equally indispensable realms and looked askance on facile syntheses. "But much the most significant thing about my point of view at the time [*The Sceptical Biologist* and *The Great Amphibian*] ... was that I was always uncomfortable about the position of ethics. ... The explanation of this difficulty was at hand, however." He found his explanation in politics, which he saw as "nothing but the attempt to objectify the most advanced ethics in the structure of society, to enmesh the ideal ethical relations in the real world" (p. 10). In developing such a political position he followed "the lead of the philosophy which most consistently allows for the social background of our thought and being, and explains what is happening, and has for centuries been happening, to human society as the continuation of all biological evolution" (p. 11).

His socialization began with the General Strike of 1926 and matured in the face of Hitler's fascism. Typically, at the start of the strike, Needham found himself on "the wrong side," but the power of the events caused him to begin reading in socialist thought. He ended by concluding that the labour movement was the most progressive focus of social advance. He and Dorothy Needham dated their long history in left politics from this time.[27]

In an article written in 1935 Needham discussed the relationship among "Science, religion, and socialism" (1943, pp. 42–73). The article stresses the eternal validity of five faces of human experience:

26. Gary Werskey of the Science Studies Unit of the University of Edinburgh is writing a dissertation on "Socialist scientists in Britain, 1918–1941: The Visible College." Although his interest is the social origin and mature social-political positions of a very important group of British scientists, he makes several observations relevant to the development of the organismic paradigm. Werskey also draws from T. H. Kuhn in his approach. He treats Julian Huxley, J. B. S. Haldane, Lancelot Hogben, Lord Blacklett, Joseph Needham, J. D. Bernal, W. A. Wooster, C. H. Waddington, Hyman Levy, and N. W. Pirie. I would argue that political philosophy is not irrelevant to the nature of a person's scientific theory, but there is no simple causal connection.

27. The Needhams were members of Thaxted Church under Vicar Conrad Noel. This congregation nurtured Christian socialism and was extremely active in the 1930s. It had parallels in movements in France and Germany. One such group in France, centered around the journal *Esprit*, numbered among its contributors Jacques Maritain. Ironically, Maritain had studied biology for a time with Driesch.

philosophy, history, science, art, and religion. Marxists were right in criticizing the opiate of religion insofar as it was blind to oppression. But science too could become an opiate insofar as it was blind to the tragic side of life and to the irreducible numinous and worshipful dimensions of the world and of man. Needham stressed the legitimacy of the orthodox negative way to knowledge of God. The numinous— sense of the holy—could acquire new forms of expression, and perhaps the liturgical and doctrinal letter of Christianity would disappear. However, the spirit of traditional religion—the relation of love between men—would be incorporated in a future classless Marxist society. In the meantime, although difficult, it was appropriate to participate both in a traditional religious life and in progressive political action. Needham elaborated the analogy of the Kingdom of God. Poor early Christians, with the "crass simplicity" of their millennial hope for the establishment of a just and loving future society *on earth*, were the models for Needham's brand of communism. Pointing out that Marx and Engels would have been more acceptable to the early martyrs and Fathers than to nineteenth-century bourgeois Christians, Needham insisted that socialism provided the moral theology appropriate to our time. The most crucial task for science was to show how the ethics of collectivism emerges from the natural world and its evolutionary processes. The basic premise of both Needham's socialism and his Christianity was that exploitation of man by man is immoral; therefore a classless society and social ownership of the means of production are essential fruits of evolution advancing from physical particles to the future world commonwealth.

Needham came to consider nature as a series of dialectical syntheses.

> From ultimate physical particle to atom, from atom to molecule, from molecule to colloidal aggregate, from aggregate to living cell, from cell to organ, from organ to body, from animal body to social association, the series of organizational levels is complete. Nothing but energy (as we now call matter and motion) and the levels of organization (or the stabilized dialectical syntheses) at different levels have been required for the building of our world.[28]

Without denying the validity of subjective and religious experience,

28. Needham 1943, p. 15. Remarking that Marx wanted to dedicate part of *Capital* to Darwin, Needham found in the dialectic a way out of mechanism and vitalism, a way to approach history in embryology.

he also transcended the individualist bias of seeing science as a quirk of the mind. Instead it helped to reveal the construction of the progressive structure of the natural and social worlds.[29] The "as if" dodge of mechanistic materialism was unnecessary. The difference between Needham's organicism and his neomechanism was simple but critical.

> This deadlock [between mechanism and vitalism] ... was overcome when it was realized that every level of organization has its own regularities and principles, not reducible to those appropriate to lower levels of organization, nor applicable to higher levels, but at the same time in no way inscrutable or immune from scientific analysis and comprehension.[30]

Before returning to Needham's biological writings, *Order and Life* and *Biochemistry and Morphogenesis*, it would be instructive to look at a last influence on his organicism, Alfred North Whitehead (1943, pp. 178–206). Needham conceived biology under the new paradigm as a "manifestation of a great movement of modern thought which sought to base a philosophical world-view on ideas originating from biology rather than from classical physics. It fused once again what Descartes had put asunder." Not only could organic and inorganic be considered within the same coherent framework, but mind and body no longer contradicted each other. For science, organicism implied succession in time and envelopes in space. The ideas of boundaries and levels were central. Function depended on position within the whole. "Statistical regularity of fortuitous random motions is not the whole

29. The possible contradictions between dialectical and structuralist perspectives was not to come into focus until Marxist thinkers such as Lévi-Strauss wrestled with them. For the time, Marx, Engels, and Lenin offered ways beyond deadlocks in the philosophy of science for Needham. He drew from Engels's *Anti-Dühring* and *Dialectics of Nature* and Lenin's *Materialism and Empirico-Criticism*. Needham felt a bond between his work and that of organicists in the Soviet Union. From *Science at the Crossroads* (papers presented at the International Congress of the History of Science and Technology in London in 1931 by delegates from the USSR, London: Kniga) he learned of the thought of B. Zavadovsky. A second Russian, N. Koltzov, was known to him through a French publication (1935). Their rejection of the mechanism–vitalism paradigm paralleled his own. Koltzov also thought in terms of fibrils in biological organization in a way compatible with Needham's view of the material basis of fields. Unfortunately, Needham did not read Russian and was not able to follow this aspect of Russian biology, but he was sympathetic to their work and tried to direct others to it, citing it frequently in his publications.

30. 1943, p. 18. Interesting essays that depict the application of Marxism to biology and sociology are Needham's 1937 Herbert Spencer Lecture at Oxford called "Integrative levels: Revaluation of the idea of progress" in 1943, pp. 233–73, and a 1941 paper entitled "Matter, form; evolution and us."

story; there is a plan of organising relations too." Needham asserted
that Whitehead had always seen the structure of the world in terms of
envelopes and succession. He considered the basic unit to be organism
and noted that science was neither purely physical nor purely biological
but was becoming the study of organisms. Needham was impressed
with *Science and the Modern World*, but it is interesting to remember that
he did not interpret it from an organismic perspective in the *Sceptical
Biologist*. But once he was firmly operating from an organismic paradigm, Needham saw a strong ally in Whitehead. Whitehead represented
to Needham a kind of convergence of elements from Marx and Lloyd
Morgan. "Little though the philosophers of organic evolutionary
naturalism may have borrowed from one another, they march in the
same ranks" (pp. 184, 186, 194).

The primary contribution Whitehead made to Needham's organicism was his critique of the notion of simple location. Field
concepts seemed essential to adequate biological theories, and explanation in field terms abided in a willingness to deal with wholes and
position effects. Whitehead's formulations supported organismic
approaches in biology from the notion of gestalten to the use of
topographical analysis.

> According to Whitehead, all things in the world are to be con-
> ceived as modifications of conditions within time-space, extending
> throughout its whole range, but having a central focal region. . . .
> In topographic analogy . . . the influence of the thing grades off
> past successive contours . . . in every direction. The connection of
> this idea with the sort of fact we are always meeting in biology,
> namely phenomena of field character, is obvious, and today the
> concept of field is equally widespread and necessary in biology as
> in physics. [p. 197]

Just as Ross Harrison's Silliman Lectures summarized and focused
his relation to the organismic paradigm in biology, Needham's Terry
Lectures and his last great scientific books, *Order and Life* and *Biochemistry and Morphogenesis*, express his mature perspectives. It is to
these works that one must turn before leaving Joseph Needham.

Mature Perspectives

> I still think that organization patterns and relations in living things,
> integrative hierarchies never exhibited in non-living material collec-

tions, are the proper subject-matter of biological enquiry, and that the recognition of their existence is in no sense a disguised form of vitalism. I still think that biological order and organization are not just axiomatic either, but constitute a fundamental challenge to scientific explanation, and that meaning can only be brought into the natural world when we understand how successive "envelopes" or "integrative levels" are connected together, not "reducing" the coarser to the finer, the higher to the lower, nor resorting to unscientific quasiphilosophical concepts.

Joseph Needham, 1968

The plans of *Order and Life* and *Biochemistry and Morphogenesis* were quite similar, and in fact the later work, though more extensive in its coverage, repeated large sections of the Terry Lectures' argument. Needham summarized his thesis in the following paragraph:

A logical analysis for the concept of organism leads us to look for organising relations at all levels, higher and lower, coarse and fine, of the living structure. Biochemistry and morphology should, then, blend into each other instead of existing, as they tend to do, on each side of an enigmatic barrier. The chemical structure of molecules, the colloidal conditions in the cell, and the morphological patterns so arising, are inextricably connected. It is easy to find instances of the way in which organization may appear already at the chemical level. We are driven to the view that the living cell possesses as complex a set of interfaces, oriented catalysts, molecular chains, reaction vessels, etc., as the organs, tissues and other anatomical structures of the whole organism.[31]

The lecture series presented support for this argument in three parts: the nature of biological order, Needham's way of referring to the

31. 1942, p. 656. This work published in 1942 under wartime conditions had been partly written while Needham was visiting at Yale. It contained three major sections: the substrata, stimuli, and mechanisms of morphogenesis. The first part treated maturation of the egg, embryonic nutrition, and so on. Part 2 considered general concepts of causal morphology such as fields, mosaic eggs and their biochemistry, amphibian development and the basic principles of morphogenesis, and organizers and genes. Part 3 discussed dissociability of developmental processes, integration of fundamental processes, differential growth, respiration and metabolism, and finally polarity and cytoplasmic organization. A friend and former collaborator, Dr. E. J. Boell, had promised to ensure publication if anything happened to Dr. Needham traveling in wartime conditions. Later the microfilm of proofs that had been sent to Yale at each stage of correction was put on display in Sterling Library in an exhibition entitled "Making of a book in war-time."

mechanism–vitalism debate; the development of biological order, his phrase for morphogenesis; and the hierarchial continuity of biological order, a study of the problem of organic form from atom to bodily whole.

In part 1 Needham emphasized that the central problem for biology was form; form in turn meant a "time slice of a spatio-temporal entity," a phrase the biochemist borrowed from Whitehead via Woodger. The first lecture outlined his debt to Woodger and to Roux, the one contributing a philosophical and logical analysis, the other setting the frame for embryological research for two generations. Out of Entwicklungsmechanik grew a dynamic analysis of form. For Needham the task remaining was a mathematization of the form problem. Science had to remain quantitative but in an enlarged sense. "There are other systems of structure besides arithmetic, and the complex components may be very faithfully and logically dealt with on their own level."[32]

Needham devoted a large part of the First Terry Lecture to a defense of analysis in biology. He rejected the argument of physicist Niels Bohr that the indeterminancy principle had anything to do with a "thanatological limitation of biological theory."[33] Meaningful subsystems could very well be dissected out of the organism and studied under experimental conditions. The problem was selecting the appropriate subsystem, not arguing that it was possible or impossible to reach an ultimate biological atom. Needham cited D'Arcy Thompson's theory of transformations as a stimulating example of exact analysis on the biological level. The issue of reductionism was simply irrelevant, but the Marxist notion of a dialectical level was helpful. Embryology, and thus the science of form, has to deal with the origin of the qualitatively new. Dialectical analysis was a rational method of approach to such transformation.

Part 2 of the Terry Lectures described in detail the experiments of Roux and Driesch and the context within which the term *harmonious equipotential system* was introduced into embryology. After a brief

32. 1936, p. 23. Needham drew a distinction between mechnaical and mathematical in scientific explanation, a distinction he would have rejected before 1929. As he stressed in the introduction to *Biochemistry and Morphogenesis*, the old controversies of mechanical versus animistic explanation were no longer meaningful. The new program of biology was more interested in the laws of levels and the explicit connections between levels (1942, p. xv). It transcended chemical embryology in the same way that organicism went beyond neomechanism.

33. 1936, p. 33. Compare with Harrison's use of the indeterminacy analogy in biology (p. 95 above).

description of developmental mechanics in the first third of this century, Needham formulated his definition of development: "Development, then, consists of a progressive restriction of potencies by determination of the parts to pursue fixed fates. It is the opinion of many that this state of affairs can best be pictured in the manner of a series of equilibrium states."[34] He used the analogy of a series of cones with a ball on the apex of the top cone in a very unstable balance. It could be stimulated to roll down the side and reach a second precarious balance, or meta-stable state. The hierarchy of cones, and of stimuli causing the system to reach new equilibrium positions, was considered analogous to the various grades of organizers in the normal course of development. For example, an organizer of the second or third grade (Spemann's ter-minology) "has no effect upon a ball (plastic region) at a higher level of instability than that at which it normally works" (1936, p. 59). Use of the notion of successive equilibria encouraged a greater mathema-tization of development, in particular the introduction of topological models.

The phenomenon in development that had precipitated the crisis of the early twentieth century was pluripotency. Driesch had re-introduced intensive manifoldness, or entelechy, to account for observed regulation. Obviously, for Needham, the principle of regula-tion had to be entirely immanent. The theory of gradients was ad-vanced to account for "intensive manifoldness above the atomic level." Gradients were, in turn, a particular expression of the more general category of field theories. Fields were a way beyond the dead-end arguments of epigenesis and preformation. To make this characteristic of field theory clear, it is useful to look at a phenomenon, definitely critical to both Harrison and Needham, of spatial repetition of pattern in biological systems. Needham believed that the biochemical basis of pattern was paracrystalline protein patterns, the postulated material basis of biological fields. The properties of such a system could account for maintenance of pattern when mass is reduced, perpetuation of pattern when mass is increased, fusion of patterns when orientation is favorable, the heteropolar and heteroaxial nature of patterned systems, and finally observed wholeness rather than mosaicism. These items were precisely the characteristics of fields that Paul Weiss developed in

34. Ibid., p. 58. *Biochemistry and Morphogenesis*, which contains a much more adequate treatment of the history of Entwicklungsmechanik, goes into helpful detail on the origin and range of terminology emanating from work in that great tradition.

Morphodynamik and *Principles of Development*. Divisibility and stability of pattern were the key requirements. Needham spent the last thirty pages of the chapter "Deployment of biological order," as well as a major section of *Biochemistry and Morphogenesis*, discussing field theory and relating it to structured molecular aggregates in organisms. The result was an organicist resolution of the field-particle dichotomy. The section included both the justification for the evocation–individuation distinction and the theory of morphogenetic hormones, issues treated in part 1 of this chapter.

The third lecture opened with a consideration of three classes of relations in a spatial hierarchy. Woodger had pointed out that a member of such a hierarchy could be treated with respect to its membership in a particular level. It also entered into relationship with a member of the next highest level. Finally, it could be studied in its relation to members of the next lowest level—the focus of traditional experiment and analysis. However, contemporary biology must learn to resynthesize. "As time goes on, biology employs more and more of the methods of actual or conceptual synthesis, and this must be so, for it is a recognition ... that ... the relations of members to the levels above them in the hierarchy are just as important as their relations to components below" (p. 112). Hierarchial order was analogous to group theory with its mathematical envelopes. The use of set theory in organismic biology parallels its importance in dealing with complexity in other modern structuralisms.

The remainder of the last lecture focused on the effort to unravel organizing relations on the protoplasmic level, the level of molecular structure. For Needham this section was representative of proper explanations in modern biology. He first outlined advances in understanding of enzyme organization, a field in which his wife had worked for years. He then sketched F. G. Hopkins's beliefs about cell geography and the history of biochemistry at Cambridge. One advantage of contemporary biological chemistry, he felt, was access to sophisticated techniques that allowed the investigator to see into cells and molecules. X-ray crystallography was the most provocative example because it revealed molecular pattern where it had not been recognized.

The discussion of crystallography gave way naturally to a consideration of the crystal structure of animal fibers and the ubiquitous presence of fibers on various levels of biological organization. His own work on anomalous viscosity of protein solutions prepared from neurulas related to his sense of the significance of fibers in field systems. "The protein chains of the cell's web or lattice must therefore be pictured rather as connected at many points by residual valencies and relatively loose attachments, *so that they can, as it were, snap back after disarrangement. . . . We may call this 'dynamic structure'*" (1942, p. 658). Such plastic, yet definite, molecular arrangement led to the assertion that, in some sense, living systems *were* liquid crystals. The statement parallels Harrison's almost word for word. The "paracrystalline state seems the most suited to biological functions, as it combines the fluidity and diffusibility of liquid while preserving the possibilities of internal structure characteristic of crystalline solids."[35] Both Harrison and Needham were intent on accounting for the field properties of twinning, dimensionality, and regulation. Both were optimistic in the 1930s and 1940s that biologists were close to an acceptable answer to the problem of form. In fact, for Needham, the vision of collaboration among molecules was a "prefiguration of mutual collaboration of social units in maintaining patterns at far higher levels of organization" (1942, p. 677).

It remains only to sketch the degree of fulfillment of these hopes, at least those for biology, as Joseph Needham judged it from a perspective of forty years. A superficial glance shows that many contemporary biologists, avoiding field terminology, have substantially refocused discussion of the organizer. The flowering of genetics has occupied attention at the expense of study of form and pattern. But at a deeper level it is possible to argue that a convergence has been prepared. Such younger workers as Wolpert and now Crick have returned to the older questions with a fresh perspective. Even the hope that topology will

35. 1936, pp. 160–61. It is worth outlining precisely what a liquid crystal is. In a true isotropic liquid the molecules show neither orientation nor periodicity. There are several intermediate states from isotropy to solid crystal, namely the mesoforms of the paracrystalline state. In the nematic condition there is orientation but not periodicity. In the smectic state the molecules have orientation and are in equispaced planes in relation to one another. True crystals show complete orientation and three-dimensional periodicity. Needham cited a quote by J. D. Bernal in summarizing the biological importance of this range of molecular properties: "In the first place, a liquid crystal in a cell through its own structure becomes a *proto-organ* for mechanical or electrical activity. . . . Secondly . . . the oriented molecules in liquid crystals furnish an ideal medium for catalytic action, particularly of the complex type needed to account for growth and reproduction. . . . Lastly, a liquid crystal has the possibility of its own structure . . . just the property required for a degree of organization between that of the continuous substance . . . and even the simplest living cell" (ibid., pp. 161–62). In other words study of the paracrystalline state was study of the connection between levels of organization.

furnish an important key has been revived in very recent thought (Thom 1970). Since the excitement of the Theoretical Biology Club days, little advance in this direction had been made. Needham has said little about current opinions on fields, in contrast to his collaborator, Waddington, who has enriched the older work immeasurably. Instead, the biochemist-turned-historian has focused on "Organizer phenomena after four decades: A retrospect and prospect."[36]

The relevance of the organizer concept always depended on the specificity of the reactions involved. The chemical data on the organizer, or evocator, were confusing. In 1942 Needham believed that workers were all too ready to abandon the search for logical consistency and write off induction phenomena as nonspecific. But he felt it was at least certain that there existed a hierarchy of inductors, chemically identifiable, operating in normal development. Careful study over time could not fail to vindicate his claim, he asserted, and by 1968 his conviction had not substantially changed. The experimental foundation of the conviction was first of all the demonstrated difference between head and tail organizers. Spemann had investigated regional specificity in the organization center and had found that material that invaginated first ordinarily acted as head organizer, whereas material invagination last stimulated formation of posterior organs. It was possible to remove material from the dorsal lip at different times, if its normal organization function was known, and to test it under abnormal conditions. If head organizer were implanted at the head level, he obtained an induced secondary head with eyes and ear vesicles. If the same material were implanted at the host's tail level, an induced complete secondary embryo resulted, its tissues having been organized from presumptive trunk and tail ectoderm. If tail organizer were positioned at head level in the host, a complete secondary embryo was obtained. If tail material were placed at tail level, one saw only trunk and tail. No matter what the confusion about the chemical nature of the evocator, some regional difference in the organization center was inescapable. Analysis of primary induction phenomena on the vertebrate neural axis remained of central theoretical relevance.

Needham had labeled inductions by abnormal substances such as methylene blue indirect induction, or liberation of the normal evocator.

36. Joseph Needham 1968 (also appears as introduction to the 1966 reprint of *Biochemistry and Morphogenesis*).

Great experimental difficulties did not excuse discontinuing the hunt for normal inductor molecules with specific effects. Support for Needham's position came in the late 1940s from Finnish and Japanese workers who showed that inductions carried out in the newt by adult tissues such as liver and kidney gave qualitatively varied responses. Some test tissues gave primarily forebrain development, some yielded hindbrain structures, and so on. Needham regarded this work as the third significant phase of study of the organizer. The first was the 1932 discovery that the neural inductor effect was stable to physicochemical denaturing procedures, leading Needham to think in endocrinological terms. The second had been Holtfreter's (1933–34) demonstrations of the release of the masked organizer from unusual tissues, including the ventral ectoderm.

Toivonen in Finland was also responsible for the fourth phase of work on organizer specificity. In 1953 he found that alcohol-denatured bone marrow induced only mesodermal structures in the newt embryo hosts. They included blood, pronephros, myotomes, and notochord; there was not so much as a single neural cell, much less structure. Somewhat earlier the Japanese school of Fujii and Okada had obtained weak, exclusive mesodermal inductions with amphibian skin. For both groups if the mesohormic extracts were heat denatured, they became neural inductors. It would be hard to reconcile these results with the hypothesis of an unspecific stimulus and leave specificity entirely to the reacting system. The hope inspired by the discovery of such effects was the eventual synthesis or reconstruction of an embryo by combining the action of particular inductors on competent tissue. The Finns and the Japanese both produced such syncretistic wholes.

However, the chemical characterization of the inductors remains confusing. Yamada Tuneo had fractionated active proteins obtained from heterogeneous tissues that gave regionally specific inductions, but the work of Hayashi Yujiro and Takata Kenzo seemed to indicate the active fraction to be the ribonucleoproteins. A modern German school led by H. Tiedemann has employed methods of high resolving power, such as chromotography, that were unavailable to the previous generation and has tested many fractions for germ-layer specific activity. Suffice it to say that the final answer to the organizer problem is not known, but the problem is hardly a false one. It would be most difficult to interpret modern practical and theoretical work apart from that of the generation of the 1930s.

Needham sees a split in contemporary developmental biology that
must be bridged, much as that between chemical and morphological
embryology in his own active biochemical period had to be spanned.
The contending schools could be referred to as reaction mechanists
versus champions of multiple specific "hormones." In significant respects the two aspects parallel field–particle problems in the 1930s.
It is not illogical to think their resolution too will be founded on an
organicist understanding of the developing embryo.

5

Paul Weiss

Omnis organisatio ex organisatione

Paul Weiss, 1940

This, then, concludes my argument. If nature were atomized and inherently chaotic, only creative mind could see and carve into it and from it those patterns of higher order to which we concede consistency and beauty. But nature is not atomized. Its patterning is inherent and primary, and the order underlying beauty is demonstrably there; what is more, human mind can perceive it only because it is itself part and parcel of that order.

Paul Weiss, 1960

From Fields to Molecular Ecology

Born in Vienna in 1898, Paul Weiss has made immense practical and theoretical contributions to the study of genesis; his work has influenced studies in embryology, regeneration, nervous system organization, general cell biology, and ultrastructural patterning. It has been common practice to examine the nature of the organismic paradigm reflected in the work of men such as E. S. Russell, W. E. Ritter, J. C. Smuts, and J. S. Haldane and then to dismiss the importance of the paradigm to contemporary work and theory in development, if not in evolution. Molecular biology, especially molecular genetics defined within a reductionist perspective, is seen as the solid foundation of current thought. Yet Weiss himself early helped spin out another strand of molecular biology, the strand that united his work to that of Ross Harrison and Joseph Needham. It is a strand that has woven together threads of particle and field explanations into a fabric of modern developmental theory defined within an organismic perspective.[1]

1. For a brief autobiographical statement and summary of Paul Weiss's work see his article

In contrast to Needham, Weiss was committed to organicism from his earliest work. In the 1920s Weiss, trained in engineering as well as biology, was thinking in terms of systems rather than stereotyped mechanisms. His dissertation, based on experiments performed in 1921, was an attack on the theory of tropisms developed by Jacques Loeb (Weiss 1925*b*). Weiss was forging himself an alternative to the mechanistic paradigm and its metaphors. The theory of tropisms was closely related to the belief that biology could be understood entirely through reduction to physics and chemistry, that is, a microdeterministic physics and chemistry. Weiss felt that as a result many explanations of biological phenomena were "nothing but translations of descriptions of facts into *inorganic terminology;* the wish has become the father to the thought" (1925*b*, p. 1). A return to a more biological way of thinking and expression was crucial to true explanation. Far from departing from the ideal of scientific exactness, he emphasized, such a program could only make explicit the coherent laws of organization of the organism and its behavior. This was also the belief of Needham and Harrison.

The basic assumption of Loeb's doctrine was that a like result must imply a like causal chain: there exists a rigid material mechanism, which when completely revealed, would make possible strict prediction of every aspect of animal behavior. Furthermore, the relevant level of the animal was the chemical level. In his thesis work Weiss tested these assumptions by studying the resting behavior of fatigued butterflies. His first experimental effort concentrated on the same class of phenomena that had provided ammunition to mechanists such as Loeb. The first long theoretical section of the dissertation justified introducing systems to replace tropisms. He countered Loeb's doctrine by insisting

---

in Galbiani 1967, pp. 237–47. For a strong statement of the reductionist frame for viewing molecular biology, see Crick 1966. In the 1930s and 1940s it was more commonly believed that organicism, expressed for example, by reference to biological fields, was an important perspective. Then in the 1950s serious challenges were presented. Accordingly Weiss's own writings regained some of the polemical tone they showed when he felt the goad of Jacques Loeb's mechanism in 1920. It would be helpful to study the nature and roots of this later challenge because reductionism had outgrown naïve mechanism. But the thesis of this essay, that a nonvitalist organicism successfully challenged the mechanistic paradigm and its associated metaphors, remains valid. It is necessary subsequently to ask if this organicism has yielded to a reformed reductionistic approach to the organism. I do not think that it has, but a satisfactory answer would entail careful examination of work in development since 1955. A partial reply, however, will emerge from an analysis of the later work of Weiss himself.

on the relevance of scale to the organism. Organization was based on a hierarchy of envelopes. To say that the operation of a higher level is *based on* the proper functioning of the components of a lower is not to say the operation of the higher can be *reduced to* the lower. Rather, the higher complex is given as a *unit* that requires its own laws. The distinction is the same as that made years later by Polanyi: boundary conditions left open by processes of a more elementary level are determined by the organizational plan of the next order. Thus there may be more variability in each component of a whole than exists in the behavior of the system itself; in this sense the whole is more than the sum of its parts. Moreover, similar reactions or animal functions do not imply identical mechanisms, but rather "mechanism ... is subordinated to the law which rules the complex as a unit. ... An explanation is only complete if it covers mechanism and meaning."[2]

A system was defined as a unitary complex that tends to preserve its state in the face of external disturbance. Variation in parts is not inconsistent with maintenance of the whole; regulation and adaptation are expected. Weiss described several examples of physical systems, such as the heating of a thermocouple, which produces an electric current tending to cool the system. The systems concept bridged the gap between organic and inorganic, a goal of Loeb, by a different route. Weiss's examples of equilibrium systems were constructed in such a way as "to lessen the intellectual discomfort which some biologists experience when they are confronted with lawful behavior not operating through the familiar 'ultimate elements.'"[3]

2. 1925*b*, pp. 2–3. Both Weiss and Polanyi believe that the idea of a machine itself makes nonsense of the reductionist philosophy of science. Weiss's example is that a drilling machine is not such a thing because of its particular structure but because its structure permits its function, drilling. Many mechanisms would serve. Polanyi and Weiss currently participate in a sort of paradigm community known as the Frensham group, sponsored by the van Leer Foundation. The group believes in the applicability of systems theory to social and human problems. Polanyi's arguments have been directed to the generations of reductionists after Loeb, those trained as biophysicists and molecular biologists, but the basic logical form of the argument is similar. Weiss's later polemics against reductionist molecular biology are aimed at the same targets as Polanyi's.

3. Ibid., p. 7. Today the systems concept is banally familiar. That was not the case in biology in 1922, when the dissertation was written. Without doubt Weiss was one of the originators of systems thinking in biology. That its applications in retrospect seem obvious does not change the fact that at the time Weiss was challenging orthodox opinion. Weiss drew on his training in engineering in his formulation of systems theory. Although he cited Köhler's work and recognized the affinity of Gestalt and field concepts, he did not get his organicism from Köhler. Weiss felt that several workers in the Gestalt school were primarily influenced not by physics

Weiss did not deny that simple reflex reactions and associated rigid structures occurred in organisms. He merely denied that they were the dominant form of organization. More interesting were the plastic reactions he found in his butterflies, whose variations in parts did not preclude a general integrated character of the whole. A characteristic series of reactions led to the fatigued animals' adopting a sleeping posture, defined in relation to light and gravity. The reaction was divided into three parts; each rigidly followed the previous component, but each phase was plastic within itself. The entire performance represented an instinct assembled from nonunitary parts. The researcher's task was to probe the dynamics of similar situations to understand physiological conditions of the animal, not to look for stereotyped mechanisms alike in all cases. So by the conclusion of his dissertation, Weiss had stated intellectual commitments that echoed throughout his later work. Details and the targets of his polemics changed, and the concepts acquired rich concrete meaning. But as Weiss turned from animal behavior to developmental biology, the components of his organicism were clearly elaborated.

It would be appropriate to explore Paul Weiss's experimental work in five sections: problems relating to the nervous system, tissue culture systems, regeneration phenomena, general cell biology, and aspects of fiber properties in biological organization. There is considerable overlap among the sections, but there is at least a rough chronological progression. The qualities of his organicism should emerge from a careful consideration of his actual experiments and the metaphors he employed to interpret them. Subsequently, it should be useful to look more directly at his theoretical speculations, particularly those relating to fields, growth control, molecular specificity, and emergent organization and self-assembly in biological systems. Finally, a consideration of a recent paper should summarize his mature perspectives on his own work. The types of paradigm links to Needham and especially Harrison will be explored, culminating in a glance at a current paradigm community in many ways like the Theoretical Biology Club.

---

but by biology, especially by regulatory phenomena. The friends later diverged in their work when Weiss decided that the psychologist relied too heavily on physics, especially electrical analogies, whereas more "biological" thinking was needed. They had met in 1927, when Weiss worked at the Kaiser Wilhelm Institute in Berlin, but they had corresponded before that time. Another early systems thinker, Ludwig von Bertalanffy, was early influenced by Weiss. He visited Weiss in 1922 in Vienna, where the two men talked intensely about the new frameworks for biology (interview in New York with Professor Weiss, August 1970).

Drawing from experiments begun in 1921 and continuing for years, Weiss concluded that the relationship between the central nervous system and sense organs and muscles could not be based on typical structural connections of an innate pattern, but that a high degree of specificity in the relationships was nonetheless indisputable.[4] The first experiments involved transplanting mature whole limbs of larvae of *Salamandra maculosa*. Later, *Amblystoma* individuals were used. The transplants were grafted into the vicinity of a normal limb to ensure innervation from the limb plexus, but at a sufficient distance to allow complete mechanical independence. Various orientations of the grafted limbs were tested for functional properties. Innervation for the grafts did not come from new sprouts from the central system but from branching nerve fibers of the plexus. After some weeks the grafts regained complete mobility. The movement showed the traits of what Weiss called homologous response; that is, each muscle of the transplant contracted at exactly the same time and with the same intensity as the muscle of the same name in the normal limb, whether or not the response was functionally adaptive. The phenomenon was observed in hundreds of cases in many combinations. If the original and transplanted limb were on the same side and similarly oriented, homologous response resulted in synchronous movement, like oars on a racing craft. If the limbs were of opposite laterality and placed dorsodorsally (Harrison's terminology), homologous response meant that elbow flexion in one limb was invariably accompanied by the same muscle contraction in the other extremity. Obviously, such mirror-image movements were detrimental to the organisms, but no learning took place. As many as three limbs, thus two supernumerary limbs, would show homologous response. A hind limb transplanted in the forelimb region showed contraction of the appropriate homologous muscle too, thus confirming by direct biological test the legitimacy of anatomical and evolutionary naming practices. Fragments of limbs were tested with similar results. Even single transplanted muscles gave correlated response movements. Weiss transplanted limbs between different species of salamanders (heteroplastic grafting) with corresponding

4. Weiss 1936. Earlier reviews appeared in 1928, 1929, and 1931 and Weiss published dozens of papers on homologous response, modulation, and resonance. I will, however, draw from only a few papers to summarize the general direction of this work and its relation to the organismic paradigm. All the elementary work on this topic, begun in Austria and continued in Germany and the United States, was completed by the early 1940s.

results. Detwiler, a former student of Harrison with whom Weiss had had some heated disputes earlier, obtained essentially the same response when he transplanted embryonic limb buds that developed into the supernumerary appendages. Homologous response occurred in all these tests only if the limbs were innervated from the same spinal region, but it was irrelevant which nerves within the region innervated the transplants. The situation was reminiscent of other harmonious equipotential systems.

Homologous response was also observed in the sensory field; centers identified afferent messages coming from muscles in abnormal locations. This conclusion was reached by observing myotactic reflexes in supernumerary limbs. When stretched, some muscles receive a reflex impulse to contract from the central system. If muscle A of a supernumerary limb were passively stretched, muscle A' of the original limb contracted. The myotactic, or proprioceptive, reflex remained the only sensory system from 1930 to 1942 for which homologous response had been confirmed. Then, with the cooperation of *Triturus torosus*, Weiss chose the lid-closure reflex, elicited when the cornea was stimulated, to demonstrate that the principle held for the exteroceptive field as well. The logic of the experiments was related to the question posed by DuBois-Reymond in the nineteenth century: If acoustic and optic nerves were cross connected, would an organism hear lightning and see thunder? Weiss transplanted eyes into the auditory or nasal region of the host so that the transplant was innervated from an abnormal sensory source. The reply to DuBois-Reymond was a sharp *no*. "The results can be summarized very simply: Touch to an eye transplanted to the ear or nose region is just as effective in producing a winking response of the normal eye of the same side as is touch to the latter's own cornea" (1942, p. 137). Extensive threshold determinations with graded tactile stimuli showed that grafted and original corneas were equally responsive.

The fundamental conclusion from all this work was simple: There existed "a constitutional specificity determining the relationship ... [of center and periphery], constant and selective for each individual muscle, identical for synonomous and homologous muscles, but differing critically for different and non-homologous muscles" (1936, p. 506). Several alternative explanations could not account for the results. Sensory control was eliminated by the demonstration that animals deprived of sensory innervation gave the appropriate response. If a supernumerary limb were transplanted into the region of a deafferented but motile limb, homologous response was observed even though both limbs were totally anaesthetic. Morphological specificity was ruled out by a variety of experiments that showed nerves readily grew into strange organs by unusual paths. The requisite degree of specific direction control just did not exist. This topic will be treated more adequately when attention is turned to Weiss's work on nerve growth in tissue culture and his successful attempts to discount chemical neurotropisms as a factor in nerve specificity. Basically, he demonstrated that mechanical, not chemical, forces were sufficient to account for most observed nerve paths. Having ruled out rigid structural stereotypic relations, Weiss introduced two principles to explain his experimental results: resonance and modulation.

The resonance principle, based on the metaphor of tuning, accounted for the selective responsiveness of end and center. Weiss criticized the telephone exchange image of the nervous system for suggesting the wrong experiments and interpretations. The term *resonance* did not imply a specific mechanism any more than the term *field* implied that its basis was understood. Rather, the principle, first described in 1923, suggested the nature of the relationship so as to stimulate research founded on fruitful analogies. The term *modulation* was introduced in 1934 to designate peripheral selectivity. "It was assumed that each muscle, by virtue of its own specificity, appropriately specifies the nerve endings, converting them from indifferent into selective receivers specifically adapted to its own use" (pp. 512–13). Modulation appeared to embrace the entire motor unit, including the motor neuron. Weiss was convinced it resulted from molecular differentiation. Each muscle was subtly different biochemically; stereochemical matching replaced stereotypic linkages. Fundamentally, the form problem was placed on a molecular rather than mechanical level. The step was significant in linking field and particle because, like Harrison, Weiss believed that asymmetrical molecular arrangements were the probable material basis of field phenomena.

Modulated peripheral neurons were in contact with a central system of matching specificity. The central system contained innate dynamic patterns for motor coordination. The spinal district, for example, appeared to contain the pattern for limb activity. Weiss reasoned that "comparable to the situation in embryology, the functional districts are represented by local fields of activity, whose boundaries are maintained in a dynamic way by the mutual interference of neighboring areas" (pp. 512–13). Neither the central system itself, nor its connections with end organs, was organized like a telephone exchange. Weiss, guided by the resonance metaphor, looked not for discrete localized centers in a segment of the central action field but for dynamic conditions controlling the specific modes of activity.

Weiss saw his work as an extension of traditional embryological techniques to nervous system physiology. Using similar categories of explanation, he often emphasized the rich source of knowledge of organization promised by study of the genesis of nervous integration. If Harrison initiated neural embryology, Weiss picked up the banner enthusiastically. In a lecture delivered in 1950 he enlarged on the basic principles of explanation shared by embryology and neural physiology and clearly related his work on resonance and modulation to the organismic paradigm (1950a). The work described above consisted basically of simple recombination experiments. The method, particularly adapted to probing the part–whole issue in biology, tested the limits of coordination. Weiss defined coordination as "the orderly relation between parts engaged in a given act." Muscles operate not randomly, but in orderly groupings. "It is a basic fact of nervous function that these groupings follow a hierarchical principle" (p. 94). The hierarchical concept was the same as the one outlined in the 1925 paper on butterfly behavior. A corollary was that coordination involved different mechanisms as a function of the level of the organism being considered. One set of organized activities would set in motion activities on another level; activities on higher levels in the organism were strictly limited by number and kind of effector mechanisms on lower levels. The studies leading to the concepts of resonance and modulation were focused on one of the lowest levels of integration of locomotion, that is, on the orderly play of muscles in a limb movement, intramember coordination. The central action system had a limited inventory of movement patterns. Weiss's work indicated that specific patterns of neuron firing were innate. The patterns were not activated through rigid structures but through resonance tuning. The suggested manner of tuning was biochemical modulation, comparable to antigen–antibody interactions. The actual origin of the central scores remained obscure, but it was obvious that "all levels higher than intramember coordination operated through activation of partial mechanisms of lower order in definite and set patterns."[5] In sum, both the conceptual

5. 1950a, p. 100. In 1941 Weiss renamed homologous response myotypic response.

and experimental approaches to nervous system integration followed the same pattern as his thesis work. Hierarchy, bounded equipotential fields, variable mechanism and structure, coordination as a system— these were the keys to Weiss's organicism.[6]

Weiss's study of the nervous system was facilitated by an imaginative exploitation of tissue culture techniques. Both Ross Harrison's methodological innovation and his formulation of central problems held Weiss's attention. Even before his arrival in the United States the Austrian had studied cell movement in culture. While in Berlin at the Kaiser Wilhem Institute in Albert Fischer's laboratory, he observed that fibroblasts followed submicroscopic fibrils in their orientation. He subjected the blood plasma medium of fibroblasts to various mechanical stresses, enabling him to orient cell movements and tissue growth at will. This was Weiss's initial foray into work leading to the principle of contact guidance (1929).[7] The early experiments were continued in the Osborn Laboratory, where Weiss, supported by a Sterling fellowship, worked at the invitation of Harrison. In this work explanted nerve cells, rather than fibroblasts, were studied. Not surprisingly, the axonal tips followed submicroscopic fibrils. At this time Weiss assumed that the guiding effect was related to the fact that the orienting fibrils and the nerve ends were of the same order of magnitude. Later he would show that this relationship was not critical (1934*b*).[8]

6. For a full, late statement of Weiss's opinions on the nervous system see his article on neurogenesis in the 1955 book edited by B. Willier, P. Weiss, and V. Hamburger (pp. 346–401). Although Weiss seemed fully convinced that chemical neurotropisms played no part in nerve patterning, other careful workers, including Harrison, were more cautious. Since modulation based on biochemical differentials was not demonstrable by chemical means then, or now, Weiss insisted that the concept was not in itself an explanation of peripheral–central matching, but only a suggestion that made much more sense than any founded on specific structural frames for vague long-distance attractions. The Willier, Weiss, and Hamburger book is curious for the small place given to genetics. Weiss did not adequately integrate genetics or evolutionary theory, particularly biochemical theories of the origin of life, into his organicism. In that sense Waddington's organicism is more complete. But Weiss's primary role in introducing systems thinking into embryology accounts for his importance in concretizing the paradigm.

7. This paper was consciously related to Harrison's 1914*b* paper.

8. Weiss and Harrison had met in Munich at the Zoological Congress in 1928 (see Harrison 1934*a*). Upon his arrival at Yale in 1931, Weiss's first efforts were directed to reestablishing tissue culture studies in Osborn, although he continued his work on regeneration and on homologous response. One of the fruits of his tissue culture work was 1934*a*. In that paper he confirmed the earlier assumption that liquefaction around brain explants *in vitro* was due to the continued activity of cells of the ependymal layer. The secretions of the cells were assumed to be proteolytic enzymes.

The analysis of axonal orientation was directed against theories of chemical neurotropism, either in embryonic nerve outgrowth or in nerve regeneration. Turn-of-the-century work had established that regenerating fibers from the proximal end of a severed nerve stump traversed the wound gap and grew into the distal stump in numbers greater than expected from chance. Cajal, among many others, interpreted such growth as the result of chemotropism; "chemical agents emanating from myelin residues or from Schwann cells of the degenerating nerve stump could 'attract' nerve sprouts emerging from the proximal stump" (Weiss and Taylor 1944, p. 533). Vigorously opposing any action at a distance, Weiss directed his attention to mechanical factors, especially orientation of the matrix in which cells move. Using experiments in tissue culture, Weiss formulated the principle of contact guidance, according to which nerve fiber tips are guided in their course by contact with surrounding structures (1941).[9] The classical experimental phenomena were called the one-center and two-center effects. Localized shrinkage occurs in any intensely proliferating cell area as a result of the dehydrating effect such cells exert on surrounding colloids. If there is one center of proliferating cells, the colloidal network is automatically distorted into a radially symmetrical pattern. "Subsequent nerve growth, being guided over these radial pathways toward the center, naturally will give the illusion of having been 'attracted' by it. . . . The one-center effect . . . is a concrete example of one way in which localized chemical activity can translate itself into structured patterns" (Willier, Weiss, and Hamburger 1955, p. 354). In the presence of two proliferating centers, the intermediate fibrous matrix is stretched between the foci, thus aligning the fibers in a straight tract. Subsequent nerve outgrowth follows the path to form a nerve bundle.

9. The extension of the observations (guidance of sprouts by fibrous stuctures of their surroundings) in culture to the living organism was reported first in a 1943 paper by A. C. Taylor, a long-term friend and collaborator of Weiss. Serveral of the many joint papers they published on nerve regeneration were related to surgical nerve repair, a topic that became crucial during World War II. Having gone to the University of Chicago in 1933, Weiss worked throughout much of the war on topics of practical importance to the wounded, and consequently he has strong opinions on the close relationship of basic research and medical application. Using his basic knowledge of cell guidance, he and his collaborators developed a technique of splicing severed nerves with arterial cuffs. The method led to the use of freeze-dried nerve stumps, blood vessels, and corneas for surgical grafting—the origin of the first tissue banks. Discovery of neuroplasmic flow also derived from the so-called applied research. This topic of basic biology will be discussed below.

Weiss stressed that contact guidance was not a crude mechanical phenomenon and that factors in nerve orientation were complex. For example, he recognized that different kinds of nerve fibers in the organism tend to follow different pathway systems when faced with a choice, revealing a measure of selectivity in contact guidance perhaps based on biochemical differentials in contact surfaces of the pathways. However, Weiss was certain that no long-range chemotropisms were involved.

Using the rat, Weiss and Taylor expanded the critique of the theory of neurotropisms by devising experiments as close to Cajal's as possible in order finally to silence the critics of contact guidance. Nerves in the rat were permitted to regenerate into forced arteries that confronted the outgrowing fiber with alternate paths. Some of the branches led into channels that contained degenerating nerve, tendon, or fatty tissue; some led into blind pouches. Observation confirmed that fibers grew into both types of channels in equal density; no preferential growth occurred into channels with alleged attractant tissues (degenerating nerve). Also, nerves approaching the entry to a channel showed no tendency to converge upon it (Weiss and Taylor 1944, p. 256).

In an article that fittingly appeared in the centennial issue of Harrison's *Journal of Experimental Zoology*, Weiss published a valuable treatment of work related to nerve repair that he had begun years earlier. The work illuminated the mechanism of contact guidance by modifying the earlier assumptions on the role of extracellular colloids and environmental surfaces (1945).[10] The basic new observation was that a cell exudate assumed to be related to collagen, "filoform protein molecules aggregated into fibrillar chains," formed an intermediary noncellular film between migrating individuals from explants and solid surfaces. The exudate was first seen in silver-impregnated preparations, but Weiss carefully ruled out the role of fixation artifact. The exudate, or ground mat, was strictly confined to a certain radius from the explant. It had a reticulated appearance, and the terminal cell filopodia always coincided with the fibrils of the mat, which reached a maximum diameter of 0.0005 mm. Advancing tips of cells were never seen to extend beyond the limits of the ground mat. The colloidal exudate seemed to join "the living units enmeshed in it into a common fabric and also [to] bind them to the substratum. It thus confers upon what

10. The paper summarized study of almost "5,000 tissue cultures, including 376 experiments specifically designed to analyze the response of cells and axons to different substrata" (p. 353).

otherwise would be isolated units, the character of a coherent tissue" (p. 337).

Exudates were studied in liquid media and clotted cultures, on scratched glass grooves, glass fibers, and textile fibers. Orientation of exudate fibrils was determined by the direction in which the mat spread. Tension, such as capillary action along a groove, resulted in oriented paths. Long cylindrical fibers generated similar forces; tips followed the long axis of cylinders whose diameter was far too large to exert any direct guiding effect. Advancing filopodia did not circle such rods. Rate of cell advance was related to the organization of the surface, a fact with important implications for nerve repair *in vivo*. For example, cells proceeded more than twice as fast and as far along the interface between a glass fiber and surrounding plasma clot than they did inside the clot. The frequent confusing intersections in the clot accounted for the delay. The ground mat phenomena clarified "mechanisms of 'thigmotaxis' or 'stereotropism' of tissue formation; and have a wider morphogenetic significance of fibrous exudates in development and wound healing" (p. 384).

Weiss interpreted his experiments in an intriguing manner. Within the fabric metaphor he focused on the forces integrating organized elements, cells, into coherent wholes, tissue patterns. The tissue behaved as a unit. Such an explanation was antithetical to the concept of tropisms acting through "individualistic" cell reactions. Weiss speculated that the ground mat mechanism might well suggest the function of colloidal surface coats in general. The work also indicates why cell surface studies have been so important to the organismic paradigm in biology: They are an investigation of organizational laws welding units into higher order patterns.

In another paper Weiss stressed that contact guidance was a necessary, but not sufficient, condition of nerve orientation (1950c).[11] The experiments involved isolating specific parts of the nervous system, and other tissues such as heart, in a nutritionally favorable but otherwise indifferent site in a larval host. The fragments of the nervous system of urodeles were provided with peripheral effector organs similarly isolated in the dorsal fin's fibrous matrix. Parts of brain and spinal cord were analyzed in relation to limbs, eyes, heart, or intestine. The results were summarized with reference to nerve outgrowth, orientation, and ter-

---

11. The experiments were begun in 1939, but publication was delayed by the war.

minal connection. The pioneering fibers followed the fibrous matrix of the fin connective tissue. If those fibers were aligned, they followed a direct path to the isolated end organ. Also, "nerves form by accretion around pioneering fibers which have succeeded in making terminal connections. This process has been termed 'fasiculation'" (p. 457). Weiss felt that formation of connecting nerves involved the two processes, orientation by contact guidance and fasiculation, with the mechanism of the latter remaining obscure.

The deplantation experiments were intended also to elucidate specificity of peripheral–central connections. It was known that sensory fibers connected only with sensory end organs, and motor fibers with motor end organs. Such differentials, Weiss reasoned, might be explained by his theory of modulation, or biochemical specificity. The experiments in the 1950 paper, however, showed that intracentral neurons did not possess such discriminatory ability but formed anatomical connections with either skin or muscle elements.

Study of contact guidance and fasiculation comprised only one component of Weiss's attention to nerve repair and embryonic outgrowth. This component involved development of the tissue-fabric metaphor and appreciation of emergent organization and part–whole relationships. The second principal element of his interest in nerve regeneration concentrated on the mechanism of actual axon growth. Knowledge of the mechanism of protoplasmic increase in nerve fibers would lead to consideration of the structure or protoplasm. Again Weiss used organismic images, similar to the paracrystalline structures of Needham and Weiss, in interpreting his experiments. The nerve enlargement work grew out of the splicing technique used during the war in surgical repair. Some of the arterial cuffs tightly constricted the enclosed nerve portion. Constricted nerves developed chronic proximal swellings and distal shrinkages. The effect confirmed that axoplasm was manufactured in the cell body and actively transported peripherally. The supposedly resting nerve cell proved to be a most active center of macromolecular synthesis. In the course of analyzing the dynamics of neuroplasmic flow Weiss once more was responsible for a major concretization of the organismic paradigm.

A paper published with H. B. Hiscoe in 1948 (Weiss and Hiscoe) summarized the significant work on nerve enlargement carried out since 1943. The experimental observations, mostly on constricted nerves of rats, showed that nerve fibers that had regenerated through a dammed zone were permanently narrowed distal to the constriction. A permanent surplus of axoplasm remained trapped immediately proximal to the constriction, resulting in ballooning, telescoping, beading—all subsumed under the term *damming*. The damming graded off proximally in a linear fashion, presumably due to increased resistance to axoplasm movement by the reduced cross section of its channel. Intensity of damming increased with time and was directly related to the degree of reduction of cross section. Drawing from a variety of observations, Weiss concluded that the configurations produced in the living fiber by damming were not caused by simple mechanical deformation but by the buildup of axoplasm produced proximally. When constricted fibers were released, the surplus axoplasm flowed, thereby widening the distal portion of nerve by about 1 mm per day, which was assumed to be the rate of normal axoplasm convection in intact nerves. Weiss found that the rate was of the same order as the required rate of protein replacement in the fiber based on calculations from known values of ammonia production in the tissue. Thus the axoplasm transported was composed of protein macromolecules needed to replace catabolized material.

The authors concluded that growth and centrifugal transport were not confined to the embryonic period but occurred continuously in the living nerve. Furthermore, the only source of the material was the nucleated cell body. This conclusion was an additional refinement of the nerve cell doctrine so crucial to Harrison's analysis of axon extension in 1907 and earlier. Distal atrophy and proximal swelling were the conclusive pieces of evidence. Damming, especially, ruled out the alternate interpretation that only an accessory factor was prevented from traveling distally where actual synthesis of protoplasm might normally take place. Weiss was firm that macromolecular synthesis in the neuron occurred exclusively in the nucleated center. To explain the deformities he postulated a dynamic pressure mechanism producing peristaltic-like waves that proceeded proximodistally. The problem of neuroplasmic flow resulted in an analysis of protoplasmic structure treated in terms of a partially plastic, partially rigid colloidal material.

> The primary object is evidently the relatively coherent matrix of the axon, which has some degree of form stability. This does not imply absolute rigidity. . . . On the contrary, its stability must be considered as of statistical nature, with mechanical links being

dissolved and reformed continually. [Weiss and Hiscoe 1948, p. 383]

Further study of neuroplasmic flow involved considerable methodological sophistication. For example, Weiss and co-workers were among the first to use isotopes from the Chicago Atomic Pile to determine that part of the swelling could be attributed to interference with a fast(i.e., faster than the 1-mm-per-day macromolecular transport), continuous stream of interstitial fluid between the actual nerve fibers. Isotope experiments confirmed that most of the damming effects were due to blocking of the slow flow of axoplasm within the fibers. Eventually, electron microscopic studies added weight to the initial conclusion.

> The nerve cell body is engaged in continuous reproduction of its macromolecular mass, foremost protein, which is then passed on to a conveyor-like mechanism of the nerve fiber channel for shipment to sites of internal consumption and repair, as well as for export of some products to extra-nervous tissue. My double training in biology and engineering has undoubtedly predisposed me to recognize and interpret correctly this 'neuroplasmic flow' and its role in the adaptive functioning of the nervous system.[12]

From the beginning Weiss's interests in developmental biology extended beyond nervous integration. Before exploring his contributions to cell biology and their relevance to his organicism, a brief glance at his forays into amphibian limb regeneration will set the stage. Weiss regarded regeneration phenomena as intrinsic to developmental concerns: "They are fundamentally of the same nature and follow the same principles as the ontogenetic processes."[13] He regarded regenerative capacity as the residue of original powers of growth, organization, and differentiation—a residue offering unique possibilities for probing basic processes. One of the first problems that attracted him was the origin of material in the regeneration blastema

---

12. Weiss, in Galbiani 1967, p. 241. Weiss's fusion of engineering concepts to those of developmental biology was definitely a constant factor in his organicism.

13. 1939, p. 458. Weiss wrote to Harrison on February 11, 1939, asking the Yale embryologist to write the foreword for his book. Because of a pressing schedule Harrison was unable to help, but he enthusiastically encouraged the endeavor. In his letter Weiss stressed that the purpose of his *Principles* was to stimulate new research, not to review systematically the past. The organismic framework of the text had a frank didactic intention (Harrison Archives, Sterling Library, box 34).

in urodele limbs. Did the animal keep a reserve supply of totipotent cells, or could already differentiated cells reorganize themselves when presented with altered conditions? In 1925 he determined that although when only bone is removed from a limb no bone regeneration occurs, if the distal portion above the elbow is amputated from a boneless limb, the new distal portion is equipped with a typical skeleton. The new bone could not possibly have been provided from the distant bone source in the pectoral girdle. The new bone came from the blastema. Analogous experiments with other tissues yielded analogous results (1925a; see also 1930). The lesson was "that the blastema is not an assortment of differentiated cells collected from independent contributions of the old tissues but a mass of *equivalent* cells which later differentiate in different directions" (Galbiani, p. 464). Once again his prejudice against independently acting elements surfaced; he saw the organism as a whole made up of overlapping, dynamically maintained field systems. The regeneration blastema was only one more equipotential system:

> The fact that the blastema is simply an organized herd of cells raises the question of how this mass acquires the definite organization necessary to build a typical organ. On the whole, a regeneration blastema can be compared to an embryonic organ rudiment. In both cases, the equipotential character of the cells can be demonstrated by the same methods. ... The differentiation of a limb regenerate is directed by the limb field of the stump. As in ontogeny, the limb field is a property of the field district as a whole and should not be associated with any particular discrete groups of elements. [pp. 470–71]

Weiss performed a variety of regeneration experiments in the years before his visit to Yale, but the above sufficiently represents the substance of his thought.

After World War II Weiss attended ever more to general cell biology, especially to mechanisms of movement, orientation, shape, and selective contact of cells—individually, in artificial groupings, and within the organism. This work forms the fourth major body of experimental concerns to be sketched in this book.

One of the first systems to draw Weiss's attention was the differentiation of cartilage of specific shape. In a 1940 paper he analyzed the role of mechanical stress factors in the formation of the architecture of the chick eye's cartilaginous sclera (Weiss and Amprino 1940). The authors also studied the time of fate determinations. Mesenchyme cells of the eye put into culture before the fourth day of incubation grow as ordinary fibroblasts, showing no tendency to develop typical cartilage. Cells explanted on or after the fourth day produce typical scleral cartilage at the same rate as in the intact embryo, construction being complete by the seventh day. Clearly, "the changes occurring in an embryonic field which lead to this gradual fixation and which are commonly referred to as 'determination,' antedate the appearance of manifest differentiation" (p. 254). Weiss believed that ever more sensitive physical and chemical means of revealing subtle molecular arrangements, perhaps in surface membranes of the cell, would illuminate previsible or implicit differentiation.

Significantly, the cartilage produced *in vitro* was not merely cartilage in the general histological sense but had actually elaborated typical morphological traits of sclera. The physical conditions of the culture medium were evidently capable of supporting development of tissue architecture, giving the biologist a most valuable test system. The successful mesenchyme cells were grown in a plasma clot. If the clot were subjected to slightly greater tensions, the scleral plate was thinner; the greater the tensions, the thinner the cartilage. Excessively great mechanical stress suppressed scleral differentiation. Both the internal cell and fiber architecture of bent cartilage revealed molding effects of mechanical stress. Support for the conclusions based on *in vitro* cases came from observations of embryonic eyes *in situ*. Eyes caused to collapse by pricking on the fourth day had thicker than normal scleras, owing to the absence of tension normally exerted by the growing bulb.

Years later Weiss returned to an analysis of cartilage development. He worked with Aron Moscona, who had carried out in Weiss's laboratory an important series of experiments on type-specific sorting out of dissociated cells (1958).[14] Study of the genesis of the architecture of a tissue is a cardinal element of the form problem, and once again Weiss searched out the concrete content of the organismic paradigm.

14. In 1952 Moscona had developed the trypsin method of cell dissociation so valuable to workers in the field in the late 1950s and early 1960s. Weiss includes a number of Moscona's publications in his own bibliography since they were so germane to his concerns and since they were often the result of collaboration. Weiss has a bibliography of more than 300 entries, including those of collaborators in addition to Moscona.

The emergence of definite organ and tissue structure during development implies that the component units ... assume patterned space relations. These reveal themselves in geometric features of position, proportion, orientation.... The ordering processes involved are variously referred to as 'organization', ... 'field action', and the like.

But terms such as *field* and *organization* were not explanations in themselves. Weiss constantly stressed that fact and saw his study of chondrogenesis as a probe of the biotechnology that underlay field processes. The net of development had to be resolved into component processes if words such as *field* were not to be an excuse for analysis. "The following report offers a small contribution to such a programme, as applied to the problem of 'tissue architecture'; specifically, the architecture of cartilage as a prototype of a structurally simple tissue" (p. 238).

In the experiments precartilaginous blastemas of chick limb buds (3–4 days) and chick scleral rudiments (6–7 days) were trypsin dissociated. The cells of each type were allowed to settle and reassociate in liquid culture. The new cell clumps were then cultured on plasma clots. Both kinds of cells developed into true cartilage, but each developed into a specific architectural variety according to the *in vivo* pattern. Both internal and external tissue structure was specific. Weiss and Moscona concluded that different cell types were endowed with "distinctive morphogenetic properties determining the particular patterns of cell grouping, proliferation, and deposition of ground substance which, in due course, lead to the development of a cartilage of a distinctive and typical shape" (p. 242). Dissociated individual cells reassociated with one another clearly possessed the capacity to reconstitute highly specific fields.

Whatever this remarkable property be, it cannot manifest itself, of course, in single cells and is evidently a group phenomenon. A single cell can form neither a plate nor a whorl. The property in question, therefore, must be of a sort that would enable the individual cells, when they join together with others equally endowed, to execute collectively a group operation of a higher degree of order. Supracellular self-ordering processes of this kind conform to the original definition of "field" effects.

Weiss thought his results confirmed, in a purely formal sense without regard to mechanism, some of Child's principles of morphogenesis. Weiss's experiments did not reveal a particular mechanism, but they did permit reconstitution of a very simple field phenomenon *in vitro*, where future study of mechanism might be particularly fruitful. "The next step should be to detect more elementary differences in behavior of cells which preferentially form plates *versus* cells which tend to form lumps: differences in aggregation, in mutual orientation, in proliferative pattern, and perhaps in fine structural characteristics of their secreted ground substances" (p. 243).

Reference to ground substance was followed by speculation that cartilage formation might be related to the pseudocrystalline organization of extracellular fabrics, such as the basement lamella of larval amphibian skin that Weiss had studied. The authors observed that "it is not implausible to conjecture that the ground substance of the cartilage may likewise play a unifying and structure-determining role, the cells thus generating an ordered matrix, to the ordering influences of which they themselves would then reciprocally submit" (p. 244). The constant organismic theme that form problems may be properly analogized to crystalline or paracrystalline processes recurs in Weiss. The cartilage system appeared to provide a most promising clue to the puzzle of emergent organization.

Earlier in another system Weiss, with Gert Andres, had approached the problem of reassociation and self-ordering into higher order complexes (1952).[15] They postulated that cell-specific aggregation phenomena "constitute an important mechanism to insure the correct assemblage of the composite body mosaic despite its great complexity" (p. 450). The problem related to the study of form on a molecular level. Weiss speculated that discriminating cell contact might well be based on subtle stereochemical surface differences. Formation of stable contacts could set in motion a variety of far-reaching processes.

The present experiments tested the fate of trypsin-dissociated embryonic cells after random dissemination through the vascular system of another embryo. A serious methodological difficulty lay in recognizing the donor cells in the host body. Therefore, only pigment

15. The first work along this line was reported in 1949. Holtfreter conducted some of the first (except the sponge reaggregation work) serious studies of properties of cell affinity and reorganization and the relation of such properties to differentiation.

cells injected into unpigmented breeds could be followed. In 22 cases (out of 408 survivors of the experiments) definite pigment concentrations were found far from the point of initial injection. Each area of pigment had been derived from one or a few donor melanoblasts that had grown into a coherent colony. In each case the cells were lodged only in sites where the microenvironment was favorable, that is, in places where pigment cells normally belong in the donor breed.

The test system demonstrated again that dissociated cells could reconstitute a complex system and form ordered wholes in favorable circumstances. Self-organization on such a high level of order had been unsuspected and lent itself to organismic explanation where mechanistic approaches would have been strained. In a 1960 paper Weiss extended the work to another system. The results were

> unexpectedly demonstrative in proving the scope and power of . . . self-organization without instructive outside intervention. . . . They demonstrate the fact that cells which have already constituted a functional organ can, after complete isolation, dispersal, and random recombination, reconstitute that same type of organ once again, and can do so in an indifferent environment from which they could have received no cues as to how to do it.[16]

Weiss believed that he was probing what Needham would have called the phenomena of individuation rather than those of evocation: he was analyzing field properties. What embryologists had diversely called segregation, emancipation, or self-organization, Weiss considered more basic than induction, which had received the lion's share of research attention. This type of study yields analogies on a higher level to self-assembly phenomena in microtubule and virus synthesis; in all cases field and particle explanations are joined by a more concrete perception of principles of organization and assembly. Following Moscona's 1952 demonstration that cells destined to give rise to cartilage or kidney would continue their proper histogenesis in tissue culture even after having been dissociated into single cells and reassociated, Taylor and Weiss prepared single-cell suspensions from kidney, liver, and skin of 8–14-day-old embryos. They were scrambled

---

16. Weiss and Taylor 1960, p. 1177. Weiss and Taylor had conducted cinemicrographic analyses of the manner in which cells establish contact, recognize one another, and react in accordance with their respective likeness or differences. The experiments reported here were the culmination of those studies.

and recompacted by mild centrifugation, then transplanted to the chorioallantoic membrane of a host embryo. Examination after 9 days revealed that the cell clumps had given rise to complete, morphologically well-organized organs with tissue components in normal mutual relations and with correct functional activity.

Weiss had repeatedly emphasized that the next step in the study of self-organization (or constitution of a field) was an examination of the properties of single cells that made the higher level phenomena possible. The study was analogous to probing the components of functional behavior. One did not reduce the more complex to the simpler, but one had to understand the limits imposed on organization by available mechanisms. Accordingly, Weiss studied cell locomotion *in vitro* and developed a theory of cellular and subcellular motility. First, he considered why cells are polarized, how they move in one direction rather than another. It had been shown that solid surfaces were essential to cell movement, but this relationship was insufficient to account for movement in one direction rather than another. "To yield directional displacement, this random variation [due to statistically isotropic environment] must be overlaid by a persistent polar asymmetry letting one pole advance more actively than the other. With Child, one would look for the source of this asymmetry in the cellular environment" (Weiss and Scott 1963, p. 330).

These experiments successfully utilized a pH gradient to polarize cell movement. Locally applied alkalization produced local surface contractions; acidification resulted in gelation. Both effects paralyzed the sector of the cell involved; thus movement occurred in the opposite sense. But the steepness of the gradient maintained in the study was too great to be plausible for *in vivo* cell locomotion. "However, it is by no means beyond the range of plausible differentials in the microenvironment of closely clustered cells . . . thus setting up a 'field' of dynamic sequelae of inhibitions, centrifugal movements, and so forth" (p. 335). The conclusions were consistent with Weiss's belief that positive attractions played little role in cell development; rather, release from inhibitions or physical restraints permitted cell advance.

In a recent theoretical paper Weiss developed a dynamic model of cell movement based upon membrane properties in an enclosed system. The result was a sort of microperistaltic wave propagated across the cell (1964). He envisaged the cell as bounded by a typical Danielli-Davson two-layered membrane and filled with fluid under pressure, thus of low compressibility but substantial deformability. Consideration of the properties of such a structure under the influence of asymmetrical stimulation led to expectation of a polarized shift of core substance; repetitive waves would have a cumulative effect. Application to the problem of axonal flow was obvious. Basically the model proposed a way to translate the scalar properties of the molecular arrangements of a lipoprotein membrane into vectorial properties of oriented movement.[17]

Weiss's work with self-organization, and its limits, in the formation of connective tissue forms an important link with Harrison.[18] The fabric image was pivotal throughout the analysis; the macrocrystallinity metaphor gained substance here also. The basic electron microscope observations were simple. The mature form of the basement lamella of amphibian larvae displayed a remarkable degree of architectural order: it resembled plywood about 20 plies thick. Each ply was about half matrix or ground substance and half discrete parallel collagen fibers about 500 Å in diameter and with a 500–550 Å periodicity. Each ply was about 5 fibers high. Fiber orientation changed by a constant 90 degrees from one layer to the next. Thus from the surface, the membrane was an orthogonal grid. The basement membrane, coextensive with the epidermis, was not derived from epidermal cells but from fibroblasts below. This fact did not rule out the epidermis as an organiz-

17. It is unnecessary to consider all the work in cell biology that Weiss and his collaborators undertook. The major point, that is, operation according to the expectations of the organismic paradigm, has been made. But before going on, it is relevant to point out two additional kinds of experiments (see Weiss 1944). Here he discussed the morphological changes of spindle cells in culture in terms of transformation rather than true differentiative switch. "In other words, all observed transformation would merely constitute a physiological adaptation, or change of state, of a particular spindle cell ... without involving a change in basic protoplasmic constitution of that cell such as usually accompanies differentiation. Metamorphosis into macrophages would represent a case of modulation rather than differentiation in the terminology suggested by Bloom ('37) and myself ('39)" (p. 205). The terminology, although it has been effectively criticized, is relevant to Weiss's basic views on differentiation considered below. A second piece of work was based on the modulation–differentiation distinction (see Weiss and James 1955). Embryonic epidermal cells were trypsin dissociated, treated with a single exposure to excess vitamin A, and grown in culture. Metaplasia, induced by the vitamin, occurred even after single exposure. Thus, the change was termed a differentiative switch, due probably to surface changes induced by the vitamin. The system seemed to provide a method of analyzing traditional determination problems in embryology.

18. Weiss and Needham have few direct links in terms of common experimental systems; they share forms of explanation and were both among the early biologists to search out field phenomena. But Harrison is the focal point for the paradigm connections to both Weiss and Needham. For the basement membrane work, see Weiss and Ferris 1954 and 1956.

ing influence for the extracellular tissue. The whole system was an intriguing mix of factors that provided a "singularly suitable object for the study of those organizational factors residing in the body that impose a higher degree of order upon tissue components than that attainable by self-organization." The authors believed that "the stacking up of layers of different orientation is a fundamental ultramicroscopic building principle based on combining properties of the constituent elements plus some overall equilibrium conditions when they appear in groups" (Weiss and Ferris 1954, pp. 536, 538).

The electron microscope revealed only electron-dense structures. Yet the role of the unresolved interfiber matrix was also likely critical because distances between fibers were too great for intermolecular forces to account for observed regularities. Interactions of fiber and matrix seemed to constitute an organized field.

> The fibers, by virtue of their interactions with each other and with their environment, would determine a field of forces with energetically distinguished equilibrium points spaced in the indicated cubic lattice pattern. The pattern of the emergent system of higher order thus would result from the fact that the interacting units themselves have a distinctly nonrandom, patterned constitution. [1968, p. 61]

This statement focused primarily on the fibers themselves. An alternate speculation placed more emphasis on the matrix, resulting in concentration on the crystal image rather than on the fabric analogy as above.

> The resulting higher order would then be based on a property of neither the ground substance alone, nor of collagen alone, but on the fact that both systems share a fundamental steric property. This . . . would truly tie this case conceptually to the lower-order one of mineralization. . . . This later hypothesis assumes that the supposedly "hyaline" ground substance in reality possesses definite structural order analogous to "crystallinity."[19]

It mattered little which hypothesis was justified by further experiment, at least in terms of the organismic requirement of bridging the field–particle duality. Both approaches suggested explanations in terms of laws of organization in a complex whole.

After observing the intact lamella, Weiss and Ferris took electron

19. 1968, p. 61. The similarity to Harrison is evident.

microscopic pictures of reconstruction of the membrane after wounding. The sequence of events was easily determined: Epidermal cells first
migrated over and covered the wound. Fairly uniform fibers of small
size (less than 200 Å) appeared in the space between the underside of the
epidermis and the subjacent fibroblasts. These small fibers were oriented at random. Then, proceeding from the epidermal face downward, a
"wave of organization" spread over the fiber mass, straightening and
orienting its elements. The fibers became packed in the characteristic
layered structure and enlarged until they were about 500 Å in diameter.[20]

Weiss was profoundly impressed with orthogonal tissue organization
and its genesis. He frequently drew from the work in lectures and
general speculative articles, two of which will be useful here in probing
the further significance of the study of amphibian connective tissue for
the organismic paradigm (1957; 1956). Weiss was emphasizing "the
emergence of a higher-order regularity from preformed macromolecular complexes, rather than from molecular solution." The statement
placed a problem of biochemical synthesis squarely within the peri-
meter of biological form. "It is the type of principle for which we have
as yet no proper explanation in terms of lower-order events" (1957,
p. 11). The "weaving of threads into fabrics, such as we find in living
tissue" seemed to necessitate the judgment that "some sort of 'macrocrystallinity' [was] a basic property of living systems" (p. 105). The
organismic bias is unmistakable.

The compounding of higher order complexes from the interaction of
organized elements necessitated a discussion of the idea of emergence
and of the predictions that living organisms would soon be synthesized
artificially in the laboratory. The 1956 article on tissue fabrics was
printed from a lecture given at a symposium in which many examples of
stepwise synthesis from molecules to macromolecules to ordered macro-

---

20. The above summary was taken from the Weiss and Ferris 1956 paper. Another example
of orthogonal structure was found by Weiss and James (1955a). A fairly convincing mechanical
stress argument could account for the orthogonal pattern in this system; a more complex argument
was advanced for the basement lamella system. Namely, the basement membrane "fabric can
be regarded, in purely formal terms, as a sort of macrocrystal with homologous macromolecular
units at nodal points of a space lattice the major axis of which changes periodically and sharply
at right angles. It seems that closer familiarity with systems of this sort may necessitate a new
conceptual adjustment in our thinking about organic structure" (Weiss and James 1955a, p. 617).
Reference to macrocrystallinity was linked explicitly with Harrison, Astbury, and Prizbram.
The difficulty was to enrich the analogy with concrete content.

molecular systems had been presented. Weiss's own contribution involved an even more impressive situation since the elements in his case
were subcellular particles or even whole cells (1956, p. 819). To obtain
clues to the principles of organization involved, Weiss, acting from
dictates of the organismic paradigm, had turned "from the finished
fabric to the manner of its fabrication" (p. 822).[21] The analysis of
developmental processes had led to the conclusion that indeed higher
order had resulted from regrouping of organized but definitely lower-
order components. On this matter Weiss agreed with the other speakers
at the symposium who had expressed great confidence in the wide, if not
universal applicability, of the principle of self-organization. However,
at just this point, Weiss made a curious distinction that set him off from
those who predicted that living cells could be synthesized by extension
of biology's new sophisticated understanding of emergent order and its
practical implications. He stressed that the process of emergent organization, perceived for example in fabrication of the basement lamella,
had only been observed in intimate contact with living cells. That is,
the system involved a kind of chicken-and-egg problem in which all the
components had at some point a necessary connection with an *already*
organized system. *Omnis organisatio ex organisatione* (1940).

Weiss felt that an important segment of his organicist perspective
required rejection of the notion of the truly synthetic cell. In a 1963
paper entitled "The cell as unit" be elaborated the grounds of his belief
(1968, pp. 123–31). He believed strongly that once the cell was physi-
cally decomposed, verbal symbols such as organization or information
were poor tools for true reconstruction. The new reductionism, he
argued, went beyond the limits allowed by concrete knowledge of
biological systems but pretended to be well within such bounds. The
argument was ancient, but Weiss affirmed that the practical progress of
contemporary biology supported a nonreductionist verdict. He reasoned that "the true test of a consistent theory of reductionism is
whether or not an ordered unitary system . . . can, after decomposition

21. This explicit expression of a key assumption about the nature of explanation that Weiss
revealed illustrates a basic difference between the organicism of the twentieth century and that
of one of its historical cousins, Artistotle's treatment of form. Aristotle believed that the developmental process was explained by the final form; the contemporary organicist biologist considers
final form to be explained by developmental process. Weiss further elaborated: "Static form is
but the outcome of formative dynamics, and regularity in space often but the geometric record
of the sequential and rate order of the component formative processes" (1965, p. 257).

into a disordered pile of constituent parts, resurrect itself from the shambles by virtue solely of the properties inherent in the isolated pieces."[22] Weiss did not deny that some real synthesis of higher order complexes from stepwise interaction of lower order components had taken place in the laboratory, for instance the assembly of collagen fibers or of virus particles. However, he said it was illogical to jump from there to the total cell. The cell as a whole required a concept of *simultaneous* synthesis rather than stepwise processes. No component of the simultaneous system was immune to scientific understanding, but the entire unit had to be present to yield a concrete cell. Cooperative existence of all parts, instead of mere conglomeration of parts, was at issue. Life was a web, not a puzzle. "Can such interlocking systems be taken apart and put together again *stepwise*, like a machine or jigsaw puzzle, by adding one piece at a time, or is the very existence of the system as a whole predicated on the simultaneous presence and operation of all components?" (p. 125) For Weiss, the question was rhetorical.

Two key factors militated against the reductionist prediction insofar as it was based on phenomena such as the self-organization of connective tissue fabric or reconstruction of organ fields.

> The first is the qualification that in order for macromolecules to be able to congregate in higher-order patterns, they must themselves possess conforming patterns of organization . . . . We have arrived at last at a point which comes close to what might be defined as "molecular control of cellular activity," only to discover that the "controlling" molecules have themselves acquired their specifice configurations . . . by virtue of their membership in the population of an organized cell, hence under "cellular control."

The second objection concerned the unit of structure and process, another perspective required by organicism. Weiss maintained that self-assembly in a reductionist sense implies static form; it focused attention

---

22. 1968, p. 124. Weiss is claiming that the choice between reductionism and organicism in biology rests on empirical grounds. But reductionism refers to the doctrine that a theory can be translated fully into terms of a supposedly more fundamental theory, usually one drawn from physics or chemistry. Weiss tends to confuse problems of support for a theory with prior logical or metaphysical issues. Although both contemporary reductionists and neomechanists and organicists develop their views in close connection with experimental and concrete evidence, the choice of perspective is metatheoretical. Kuhn's notion of paradigm is helpful in tracing the roots and implications of such quasi-philosophical aspects of a biologist's beliefs.

only on structural features and neglected the "inseparable complementarity between *structure* and *process* in the living system, in which processed structure is but an outcome of structured processes" (pp. 126, 127).

The coordinated unity of the cell was what Weiss meant by the organismic dictum that the whole is geater than the sum of the parts. The very system character of the cell, and thus of the organism since the triumph of the cell theory, implied an all-or-none situation. Weiss insisted that the reductionist understanding of the cell still depended on an inappropriate mechanical metaphor. In particular, the structure–process dichotomy of the mechanistic approach was maintained in the new reductionism.

> The fact that diverse activities of a definite pattern can coexist . . . in the space continuum of the cell even in the absence of tight compartmentalization, reveals that although only a fraction of the cellular estate is strictly structured in a mechanical sense, there is still coordination among the diverse biochemical processes, which evidently must remain relatively segregated and localized. So here we are back again at the question asked before: Coordination by what?

For Weiss the answer was coordination by the whole. As in the many-body problem in physics, "if *a* is indispensable for both *b* and *c*, *b* for both *a* and *c*, and *c* for both *a* and *b*; no pair of them could exist without the third member of the group, hence any attempt to build up such a system by consecutive additions would break down right at the first step"(pp. 127, 130).[23]

There is no question that Weiss emphasized these doctrinal issues in reaction to the new reductionism of some molecular biologists after the impact of Watson and Crick. He seldom named his adversaries, as he did earlier with Loeb. The new reductionism was deeply rooted in genetics, especially molecular genetics, an area Weiss paid little attention to. The perspective Weiss opposed is amply treated in Crick's *Of Molecules and Men* and in J. D. Watson's *Molecular Biology of the Gene*.

---

23. The relationship of the study of the basement lamella to the traditional form problem in biology has been explicated above. But the work bore still more fruit in the understanding of form. Arrays of ribosomes in the cells in the electron micrographs of the connective tissue seemed to be in helical patterns. The suggestion was confirmed in a later paper (see Weiss and Grover 1968).

With the exception of Waddington, researchers with a basic interest in genetics have tended to ignore pattern problems, Weiss's major concern. To that extent Weiss and the new reductionists were simply talking past each other because their experimental experience led down different paths. Waddington best exemplifies the union of concerns in an organismic framework. But on significant issues, such as the molecular basis of cell organization, Weiss and his opponents were arguing differently about the same data. Here the differences were logical and philosophical. This book has noted one root of organicism in the soil of molecular biology: Weiss's study of self-organization. Stressing that the synthesis of true organisms was possible in principle from reassembly of lower order components, the reductionists were not convinced by the argument of stepwise versus simultaneous synthesis. Weiss argued that words such as *information* and *organization* were excuses for explanation; men such as Crick insisted that *fields* and *levels* were in the same boat. Weiss exposed his flank in the whole matter by maintaining that the synthetic cell would be impossible, instead of insisting that an adequate perspective on any such future achievement would have to satisfy organismic demands. He was confusing self-assembly processes with reductionism as a philosophical position. In turn, the reductionists have not met the issues raised by adoption of machine metaphors and continue to argue in philosophical categories appropriate to traditional mechanism and vitalism.

Kenneth Schaffner, defender of the modern reductionist perspective, correctly observes that both the current and past controversies hinge on the notion of organization. Ludwig von Bertalanffy defined the organismic perspective in his *Modern Theories of Deleopment* discussed above, and Weiss's views are little different. Schaffner concedes that the organismic approach to wholeness might be heuristically valuable at certain stages of biological inquiry. Several types of investigation of the organism must proceed simultaneously. But based on his survey of molecular biology (i.e., molecular genetics), Schaffner denies any evidence exists for the inherent autonomy of biology. "Moreoever since genetics occupies a central position with respect to the problem of growth and differentiation of an organism, there is evidence that these processes will eventually admit of a complete explanation" (1967). Schaffner argues that the inability of current theories of chemistry and physics to predict a unique molecular arrangement for complicated systems such as the cell is not reason for postulating autonomous biological levels of organization. The arrangement of molecular parts appears as initial conditions—field conditions—in the explanatory sentences of a biological investigation, but

> the fact that these initial conditions are not easily derived from the physico-chemical theory is not an argument against reduction. The history of the system . . . is undoubtedly a record which is explicable in terms of physico-chemical theory . . . when they are supplemented by statements describing the actions of wind, water, radiation, heat, air pressure, and so on, throughout time. To explain the system in these terms would be pragmatically impossible; consequently we take the organization of the chemical elements of the biological system as given.[p. 646]

It is ironic that the modern reductionist, as much as the former vitalist, takes organization as axiomatic, rather than as the foremost focus of thought and experiment. Needham, Weiss, and other organicists have been unimpressed. Schaffner dismisses the old warnings of Schroedinger and Delbrück that life might ultimately have to be explained by autonomous principles. In so doing, he expresses classic hopes within a mechanistic paradigm that problems refractory to immediate solution will be solved *within current frameworks* of physics and chemistry. It would be difficult to find a better expression of the position that Weiss has devoted his life to refuting.

The consideration of the five major constituents of Weiss's experimental concerns after the completion of his thesis work has led back to his dissertation's starting point: the notion of a system. At this juncture it would be profitable to explore some of Weiss's purely theoretical ideas. We begin with his field theory and general outlook on development formulated in the 1939 *Principles of Development*, glance at a treatment of growth control based on molecular specificity and at the concept of molecular ecology, and finish with an analysis of the most recent and mature formulation of his organicism. This survey should tie together the experimental and speculative sides of Weiss and reveal more clearly the paradigm links between him and other modern structuralist scientists.

The *Principles of Development* was organized into four chapters: phenomena, methods, principles, and finally development of the nervous system. The first section contained Weiss's definitions of *development* and of *organization*, the third his treatment of fields. Development, he

asserted, refers to slow, progressive changes in an organism with reference to later form and function. But it is insufficient and misleading
to regard development as preparatory to function. Rather, "we feel that
if the *actual processes* are the essential phenomena, it would be quite
beside the point to rate them according to what we surmise to be their
purpose. . . . Our prime efforts must be directed toward defining and
explaining the phenomena of nature *from their objectively demonstrable
properties*" (1939, pp. 7–8). Traditional teleological explanations had
relied on subjective ascription of goals. Organismic explanation would
look to processes coordinated into wholes in order to probe form and
function as a unit.

Weiss's treatment of the nature of organization was consistent with
his definition of development.

> This order according to which every part is put into its proper
> place, and into specific relationships with other parts, and
> according to which the activities of every part are made to comply
> with the plan of the whole system to which it belongs, is called
> organization. [p. 102 (italics removed)]

There are degrees of organization evident in nature, so the organism
must be conceived as a complex system of hierarchies of different
orders of magnitude with each level manifesting its own specific mode
of organization. The hierarchies of the organism must involve time as
well as space. Such a framework makes nonsense of the search for the
one key problem of development, be it called the genetic code, gene
control, or anything else. The task of embryology is to elucidate
mechanisms and principles in all the diversity appropriate to various
levels of integration. This view calls attention to the organismic notion
of the relation of the whole to its parts. The old either/or dichotomies
must be avoided by realizing that "an entity of any level is composed
of units of the next lower order of magnitude which are both coordinated and interrelated among one another and integrated into
the whole which collectively they constitute" (p. 109).

Either/or formulations rest on a mechanical understanding of the
organism, but, Weiss reiterates,

> organisms are systems in the full meaning of the term. . . . Briefly
> we can define it as a natural object that exists and preserves, or at
> least tends to preserve, its state and character by its own intrinsic
> forces. The converse of a system is an aggregate or pile. . . . While

one can change or remove parts of an aggregate without altering
the condition of other parts perceptibly, the parts of a system are
in such permanent interaction that whatever affects one part,
involves all others, too. The steady state of a system is determined
by the equilibrium of its forces.

All these affirmations, extremely familiar by now, are the basic
commitments of organicism. Weiss interpreted the cell theory in terms
of systems theory, a fact evident from his opinions on artificial cell
synthesis. "Gradually the emphasis placed on the individual cell as an
isolated and autonomous element dwindled, and the conception of
the organism as a system in which the individual cells assume subordinated parts gained ground" (pp. 111, 113 [italics removed]).

Within this context Weiss presented his controversial field theory.
He had first openly elaborated it in *Morphodynamik* of 1926 and its
essentials remained unchanged in the 1939 text. Weiss introduced the
concept in connection with work on regeneration and later generalized
it to ontogeny as a whole. Spemann had used the term *field* in 1924, but
he had no rigorous meaning for it. Gurwitsch had introduced the
notion into biology in 1921 as a substitute for his concept of *Morphe*.
Nonetheless, it remains true that Weiss was the originator of field
theory in embryology, both by virtue of his early commitment and by
virtue of the explicit development of his opinions. *Morphodynamik* had
introduced *fields* to name the phenomena observed in amphibian tail
bud transplantations to the limb area. If the tail bud were transplanted
early, it gave rise to a limb, not a tail, in its new location. But if "tail
determining influences" had been active for a longer time, the tail bud
produced a tail even in the limb area. Some forces present had to be
capable of organizing the indifferent cells of the bud into specific forms.
The analogy was developed to include charged and uncharged
electrical bodies. The system of organizing actions that proceeded
from an organized material to its own and foreign parts was named a
field. Fields divided into smaller fields during development until the
embryo was virtually a system of equilibrated spheres of coordinated
action.

Manifest field properties could be described, although such formulations did not pretend to explain rather than merely name the phenomena.[24] First, "field activity is invariably bound to a material

24. See the introduction of the field concept and an explanation of the status of fields for
Weiss (pp. 54–59 above).

substratum." Weiss maintained that Gurwitsch's fields did not meet this criterion. "A field is primarily an entity and not a mosaic." This property covered field pattern and self-conservation of the system. "A field district is characterized by the fact that none of its elements can be identified with any particular component of the field, although the field as a whole is a definite property of the district as a whole." The proper analogy was to the magnet. "When the mass of a field district is reduced, this does not affect the structure of the field as a whole." Size regulation had been confirmed in many experimental systems. The corollary required that a field split in half leave "each half in possession of a complete proportionate field equivalent in structure to the original field." Finally, fusion of field districts could result either in a single coherent larger field, if orientation of field axes coincided, or in two fields competing within the mass of the tissue, if orientation were improper.[25] All these properties were abundantly evident in concrete experimental systems; much of the book was taken up in extensive documentation.

The field concept defined development in dynamic instead of geographical terms. Every aspect of ontogeny had to be viewed in a double light, as the result of "interactions between the material whole with its field properties on the one hand, and the material parts on the other." Field factors themselves showed definite order: they were three-dimensional heterogeneous systems. The idea of a center, around which field intensity gradually graded off, led to the concept of field gradients. However, Weiss insisted that "field gradients are merely convenient symbols to indicate direction and rapidity of the decline of the resultant field action; as physical entities, they are just as fictitious and non-existent as is the field center" (p. 291).

The last statement foreshadowed a distinction between field energy and pattern. Field energy was related to Child's gradients of activity and tied in with the dynamic character of development. That some morphological polarities seemed to coincide with quantitative metabolic gradients, if any existed, did not imply that form was explained by Child's approach. Rather, the problem of protoplasmic structure would for Weiss, as for Needham and Harrison, prove more promising in probing the material basis of field phenomena. For Weiss, physio-

25. 1939, pp. 293–94. It is obvious that Coleridge's idea of organic form explained in chapter 2 and Weiss's treatment of field are very similar.

logical gradients were not likely causes of morphological polarity, but gradients might be necessary energetic concomitants of development. Activity gradients might indicate field phenomena and express the effects of local irritation or stimulation. Nevertheless,

> whatever the primary effect of the irritating stimulus may be . . . it has no bearing on the *pattern* of the developmental processes which follow. Although these processes may derive their *strength* from the metabolic effects of the primary stimulus, their *character* is determined by the latent formative tendencies (fields) of the irritated region. [p. 383]

Weiss's opinions on fields provide a clue to understanding his approach to the organizer problem and induction in general, a critical issue for the organismic paradigm. In one of his most insightful papers he presented his views on the organizer (1935). The organizer issue had emerged in the context of study of dependent and self-differentiation; it is impossible to overestimate the debt of embryology to Roux for the formulation of central questions. But development did not lend itself to explanation through simple dichotomies, and Weiss asserted that determination phenomena, including those of the organizer, had invited simplistic approaches. He noted that Harrison was a strong voice, in his 1933 symposium paper on determination, calling for a more adequate idea of organization. Needham too, by virtue of his insistence on the dissociability of fundamental processes in development, spoke for an appreciation of multiple formative factors. There existed no primary, privileged process.

Thus, it was suspect to reduce the organizer issue to the search for a single chemical stimulus. The grafted material had more than a simple stimulating effect; it influenced orientation and regional specificity. Therefore, the effect of the organizer graft on host tissue must involve the interaction of two systems. Appropriately, Weiss introduced his field concept at this stage to interpret the organizer and, indeed, induction in general.[26] At the conclusion of his brief interpretation of

---

26. Also at this point, Weiss defined *fields*. In most respects the definition was identical to the 1939 version, but he included in the earlier paper a specific comparison to Köhler's approach: "It is quite possible that eventually 'fields' will turn out to be merely 'systems' of specific configuration in space and of specific transformation in time [cf. Köhler 1947]. In any case, they certainly seem to comply with the rules that hold for organismic systems in general" (1935, p. 655).

the experimental corpus on the organizer, Weiss cited his basic agreement with Needham's and Waddington's evocation–individuation distinction. However, he criticized the British school for overemphasis on the evocation or chemical stimulus pole of the problem. Weiss's extremely strong field bias caused him to consider evocation trivial compared to the processes of the responding systems; he was markedly suspicious of any specific single-substance hypothesis. Thus he resisted seeing organization as merely a series of inductions. He concluded,

> in regard to the problem of organization no essential progress has been made by all these fascinating results obtained with dead inductors and extracts. The inductive principle seems to be as loosely connected with its product as the kindling spark is with the pattern of fire-works. [p. 667]

Needham would adamantly resist such a radical perspective, but it is obvious that Weiss's position on the issue was a direct result of his conception of interacting field systems.

A paper written in 1950 summarized Weiss's mature opinions on development in general (1950b). He saw growth and pattern as emergent field effects and looked to the steric properties of molecules for an understanding of differentiation, growth, contact relations of cells, induction, and protoplasmic reproduction. The general concept covering his position was molecular ecology. The unification of field and particle in the concept is perhaps its most interesting property. But before exploring molecular ecology in greater detail, it would be fitting to examine more closely Weiss's bridge between growth control and molecular specificity.

Weiss developed a mathematical model for growth control based on the notion of template and antitemplate in a system of feedback inhibition.[27] The model was not intended to prejudice mechanisms beyond the fundamental assumption that molecular form fitting was involved. Weiss conceived this speculative paper to be in the tradition of D'Arcy Thompson, the thinker so seminal for the organicist conception of form as formative process. The growth model elaborated in the paper was simply a formal scheme that might function as a working model. First a qualitative description was given, and from it Weiss and

27. Weiss and Kavanau 1957. Weiss's ideas on the specificity of growth regulations are also extensively explained in 1968, especially chapters 10, 11, and 12.

Kavanau derived a series of equations that could be shown to generate curves corresponding to empirical growth relations. The authors were careful to caution that quite different formal models could generate the same end result, but they felt theirs was a plausible approach. It clearly exhibited the traits of dynamic molecular structure within self-regulating systems that were typical of the organismic school.

The basic assumptions of the model were easily stated. Growth was defined as net gain of organic mass by a bounded living system. This mass consisted of two functionally distinct compartments, the generative component including the means of protoplasmic reproduction, and the differentiated mass, derived from the generative and made up of terminal, nonreproducing products. Each particular cell type produced its specific protoplasm in which key compounds called templates acted as catalysts. Each cell also manufactured a specific antagonist, the antitemplate, that would inhibit reproductive activity promoted by the catalysts. The antitemplate, then, functioned as a feedback inhibitor. Thus, final size was a function of an equilibrium "between the incremental and decremental growth components and of the equilibration of the intracellular and extracellular 'antitemplate' concentrations" (Weiss and Kavanau 1957, p. 44). Finally, both generative and differentiated mass were subject to metabolic degradation and replacement. Differential equations were devised and integrated to express the above interrelationships. The general solution was measured against real chick growth and found to yield reasonable values. A major test of the model was its ability to predict correctly the course of growth regulation after experimental or pathological disturbance in an organ. The model duplicated the empirical compensatory growth spurt of injured tissue as well as the temporary overshoot of the final steady state level. The oscillatory process characteristic of many feedback systems was another point of convergence of the organism and model. The template–antitemplate hypothesis was analogous to molecular form relations in immunological reactions.[28]

28. An earlier paper in the same vein as the growth model work, also conceived in the tradition of D'Arcy Thompson, reported an analysis of shape change for mesenchyme cells in quantitative terms (see Weiss and Garber 1952). The ultimate goal was to express all form changes in quantitative terms and in terms of their genesis. The authors described on a single quantative scale the various shapes assumed by chick heart fibroblasts in reaction to the fibrous texture of the medium. The fibrin concentration was systematically varied in two series, plasma concentration and pH.

Weiss believed that the role of molecular form in fundamental developmental processes extended far beyond growth regulation. Weiss began as an engineer, studied animal behavior from a systems perspective, turned to regeneration and then general embryology, cell biology, and development. He never was involved in the great current of genetics and its associated molecular biology. In fact he was often in basic disagreement with the opinions expressed by molecular geneticists about the nature of organic organization. Yet he seriously considered himself a molecular biologist, at least in certain of his perspectives and experiments. But for Weiss, molecular biology was molecular ecology, an expression he coined in 1947 (1949). He surveyed the molecular level from the standpoint of hierarchically organized systems and stressed the need to build a bridge from the organismic to the molecular level, a program shared by Needham.[29] Molecular ecology implied a statistical concept of the cell intended to describe how chemical activity transformed itself into physical and morphological structure. Weiss stated the simplest outline of the concept in a few sentences:

> Each cell and organized cell part ... consists of an array of molecular species whose densities, distributions, arrangement and groupings are determined by their mutual dependencies and interactions, as well as by the physical conditions of the space they occupy. These species range from the elementary inorganic compounds to the most complex "key" species characteristic of a given cell. Chemical segregation and localization within the cell result from molecular interplay, as only groups of elements compatible with one another and with their environment can form durable unions. [1949, p. 476]

This framework was obviously operating in Weiss's work on cell contacts and self-organization, in speculation on molecular orientation in induction phenomena and on growth regulation, and even in his early concepts of modulation in the nervous system. A system of steric

29. Weiss expressed his hierarchical perspective in an administrative reorganization he effected in the Division of Biology and Agriculture of the National Research Council in 1951. "I restructured the administrative subcategorization of 'biology,' previously based on forms of life ... or on methods of study ... by a hierarchical system of order according to functional principles in common to living organisms; to wit, in ascending order: Molecular, Cellular, Genetic, Developmental, Regulatory and Group and Environment Biology. ... This scheme of classification ... has since become rather widely applied" (1969, pp. 367–68; also in Koestler and Smythies 1969).

interlocking implied a great role for opposing surfaces in cells and organisms. Thus Weiss's considerable interest in surface properties was entirely in keeping with his organismic framework.

In a plea for research to bridge molecular and cell biology, Weiss extended the implications of his concept of molecular ecology.[30] The paper was an argument against reducing cell to molecular biology. The difference in the concept of structure for the mechanistic and organismic paradigms was plain, firmly excluding both the notion of rigid structure and of homogeneous solution. "We find ourselves right back at our initial proposition, that cellular order is based on the orderly channelling, that is, the systematic restriction of degrees of freedom, of energy distribution for the attainment of maximum efficiency." Not surprisingly, Weiss spoke of semifluid paracrystals and topographic inequalities in the cell as keys to dynamic structure. All the techniques of molecular and cell biology—the electron-microscope, the sophisticated biochemical procedures—had revealed the importance of macromolecular aggregates. "The more anisodia-metric and asymmetrical molecules are, the better, . . . they lend themselves to ordering into higher-order assemblies, either transient or permanent. In linear array, they constitute fibrils; in planar array, membranes." The most fruitful principle for the unification of study of cell and molecule was that of progressive complexification. "The inference is obvious. The bridge from molecule to cell needs a mid-stream pillar—the collective behavior of molecular populations as ordering step" (1961, pp. 107, 113, 119). The language is now eminently familiar; work within the organismic paradigm virtually required Harrison, Needham, and Weiss to turn to molecular form in resolving the structure–function dichotomy in developmental biology.

Weiss began his work with a rejection of Jacques Loeb's theory of tropisms and a development of the idea of systems. His most significant recent paper, returning to the same topic, provides a comprehensive statement of Weiss's current paradigm commitments. The essay was written to be delivered at a meeting of the Frensham group and a symposium sponsored by Arthur Koestler in Alpbach, Tirol, Austria. These meetings reflected the operation of a paradigm community like

30. 1961, "Structure as the coordinating principle in the life of the cell," in 1968, pp. 96–122. Weiss, a friend of Astbury, judged his work and opinions compatible with those of the great British crystallographer.

the Theoretical Biology Club of the 1930s. The participants included the most active organicist-structuralists in contemporary science: Jean Piaget, C. H. Waddington, Ludwig von Bertalanffy, and Paul Weiss. The roots of organicism for all these men go back to the seminal days of the late 1920s and early 1930s. It would be enlightening now to follow Weiss through his presentation to these colleagues.[31]

The Living System

$$1 + 1 \neq 2$$

Paul Weiss, 1967

Weiss's objective was to document that ancient controversies about the nature of the organism faded in the light of realistic studies of actual phenomena (1969, p. 362). He believed that the principle of hierarchical order and the necessity of regarding organisms as systems subject to network dynamics in the sense of modern systems theory were required not by a particular philosophy, but by the observed behavior of organisms. The modern updating of the mechanistic concept by introduction of the terminology of information theory did not substatially alter the deficiencies of that ancient doctrine. That Weiss did not admit his organicism to be the outgrowth of a philosophical perspective, but to be the only reasonable empirical framework for biology, is not surprising. The nature of paradigm commitment dictates that the organism must be explained by, and limited to, its lights. Weiss recalled his dissertation work and reiterated his rejection of tropisms, a theory that described the organism as a puppet pulled by environmental strings. His essential objection was that the environment too is an organism; one thinks of the impact that a similar contention, made in Henderson's *Fitness of the Environment*, had on Joseph Needham in his struggle to transcend neomechanism.

A natural organism was for Weiss a "thing" in Whitehead's sense. Parts of the universe are distinguished mentally as repetitive, patterned arrays with relatively durable form, but the real world is an irreducible

31. Weiss met Koestler when the latter sent galley proofs of his *Act of Creation* for the biologist to respond to remarks on the resonance principle. Weiss said he later persuaded Koestler to study at the Stanford "think tank" (Institute for Behavioral Studies) and was in turn persuaded to come to Alpbach. Weiss met Piaget in the 1960s but said he had long known and appreciated his work. Polanyi, another important organicist, participates in the Frensham group with Weiss. A careful study of the precise intellectual ties among all these workers would be quite instructive. It would also reveal Waddington's break from others at the meetings.

continuum; analysis inescapably is a mental abstraction. However, Weiss also stressed that synthesis is essentially abstract. One hope of science has been to arrive at a coherent description of the universe by continuous application of an additive synthetic method, but

> we are concerned with living organisms, and for those we can assert definitely and incontrovertibly, on the basis of strict empirical investigation, that sheer reversal of our prior analytic dissection of the Universe by putting the pieces together again, whether in reality or just in our minds, can yield no complete explanation of the behavior of even the most elementary living system. [p. 365]

So life is process, not substance. It involves vast numbers of dynamic structures interacting in time and space; life consists of orderly, complex, group behavior whose limits are defined by rules of order empirically unearthed. The idea of limits leads to that of levels. Appreciation of hierarchical organization remains the fundamental difference between organicism and any form of reductionism. Without the notion of hierarchy it is impossible to develop an adequate expression of wholeness because the systems concept is the embodiment of the

> experience that there are patterned processes which owe their typical configuration not to a prearranged, absoluted stereotyped, mosaic of single-tracked component preformances, but on the contrary, to the fact that the component activities have many degrees of freedom, but submit to the ordering restraints exerted on them by the integral activity of the "whole" in its patterned systems dynamics. [p. 366]

The idea of the whole as more than the sum of its parts derives from collective behavior. A system whole was operationally defined as "a rather circumscribed complex of relatively bounded phenomena, which, within those bounds, retains a relatively stationary pattern of structure in space or of sequential configuration in time despite a high degree of variability in the details of distribution and interrelations among its constituent units of lower order" (p. 369). The basic trait of a system, then, was invariance of the whole greater than the flux of the parts. Such a definition describes the exact antithesis of a classical machine. In a hierarchically organized system each subsystem controls its own subordinate parts within its own domain and in turn has its own freedom limited by the rules of order of the next higher level.

After a strong assertive presentation of his perspective, Weiss documented his case from research in contemporary biology. He detailed the functioning of cellular organelles as subsystems. Structure and process become synonymous in his conception of the cell. Form is formative process. "We encounter here the phenomenon of emergence of singularities in a dynamic system—unique points or planes— comparable, for instance, to nodal points in a vibrating string." The emergence of subpatterns is a function of the overall dynamics of the system. Weiss does not deny that a given form in a cell might arise from precisely preprogrammed steps. He maintains only that the general and primary type of formative process in the organism is the systemic one. Drawing from work on self-assembly of cilia, he sketched the theory of macrocrystallinity. The notion is essentially dualistic, uniting field and particle in the description of order on a supramolecular level. "Consequently, the acknowledgement of field continua as ordering principles in systems on the integral level is as valid and indispensable as is the practical acceptance, on the differential level, of discrete singularities within those continua, whether sub-atomic particles, atoms, molecules, molecular assemblies, organelles, cells, or cell assemblies" (pp. 379, 383). Weiss summarized his idea of biological regularity, in contrast to machine microdeterminism, as stratified determinism, macrodeterminism. He spoke of the "grain size" of determinacy in much the same way as Harrison did in discussing differentiation and orientation in the limb bud.

All the above was a prelude to Weiss's critique of the anthropomorphic reductionism of the central dogma of genetics since the exciting discovery of the role of DNA and the genetic code. Weiss was thoroughly unimpressed by use of words such as *information, control*, and *regulation* as substitutes for analysis of complex group behavior. Genes are part of the hierarchy of the organism; they interact, they do not control. Weiss developed a variety of metaphors and concluded that the proper ones for living systems are such forms as networks and fabrics, which are compatible with position and field effects. He completed his presentation by recalling that biology has made impressive advances with the help of the tools of physical science but that now it must widen its conceptual framework. For, "biology must retain the courage of its own insights into living nature" (p. 400).

Weiss has written prolifically on all these topics and more, but it would be superfluous to pursue his formulations further. His work has

shown remarkable continuity from the first discussion of systems behavior to his most recent publications. The organismic paradigm is
evident throughout. It clarifies his interests, interpretations, and
limitations—especially his extreme position on the simultaneous
functioning of subsystems of the cell, which made it difficult for him
to consider the origin of biological systems. However, both the chief
problem and tremendous power of any structuralism is the unification
of history and structure. Within the organismic paradigm Weiss
developed powerful concepts of emergence and self-organization but
faltered at the question of the origin of life. The limitation is not trivial,
but it is less striking when the context of the polemic on the cell as a
unit is remembered. Weiss felt the challenge of the new reductionistic
theories of biological organization, which had gained strength from a
genetics with little appreciation of the form and pattern problem in
biology. Weiss's organicism was strongest and most seminal for biological science in his concrete experimental work rather than in his later
polemics. His studies of resonance and modulation, contact guidance
and fasiculation, neuroplasmic flow and protoplasmic structure,
regeneration, cell sorting and organ reconstruction, and finally construction of tissue architecture in the basement lamella all express great
sophistication. All theoretical formulations—system behavior, field
organization, macrocrystallinity, growth regulation, molecular ecology
—have grown from fertile experimental soil. If Harrison pioneered in
the building of nonvitalist organicism and opened the field of neural embryology and the method of tissue culture, Weiss exploited the potential
of the paradigm in one of the richest biological careers in this century.

6

Conclusion: Of Paradigms and Scientists

The glory, doubtless, of the heavenly bodies fills us with more delight than the contemplation of these lowly things; for the sun and stars are born not, neither do they decay, but are eternal and divine. But the heavens are high and afar off, and of celestial things the knowledge that our senses give is scanty and dim. The living creatures, on the other hand, are at our door, and if we so desire it we may gain ample and certain knowledge of each and all. We take pleasure in the beauty of a statue, shall not the living fill us with delight; and all the more if in the spirit of philosophy we search for causes and recognize the evidence of design. Then will nature's purpose and her deep-seated laws be everywhere revealed, all tending in her multitudinous work to one form or another of the Beautiful.

Aristotle

The question can be postponed no longer: Did a fundamentally new way of viewing the organism appear in the early decades of this century? It is time to return to Kuhn's basic notion and reexamine Harrison, Needham, and Weiss in relation to the scientific context in which they worked. Three aspects of a paradigm have been repeatedly stressed in this essay: metaphor or model, community, and revolutionary change. Kuhn proposed the device of paradigms to explain change and growth in science, but he considered the idea of philosophical as well as historical importance. An obstacle to examining critically the relevance of the notion to any particular science, in this case developmental biology of approximately a fifty-year period, is the set of myriad meanings for the word *paradigm*. Margaret Mastermann sketches no fewer than twenty-one uses found in the first edition of *The Structure of Scientific Revolutions*; Kuhn refined and limited himself somewhat in the preface to the second edition. Despite the multiple layers of meaning, the idea of paradigm consistently points in three

substantive directions. Mastermann distinguishes the categories artefact paradigm, sociological paradigm, and metaparadigm; this book
treats the subdivisions of metaphor and model, community, and
revolution as roughly parallel. Let us review each element separately.
It would be appropriate in this context to consider several criticisms
of Kuhn's scheme as applied from these three perspectives. Next, this
chapter will return to a discussion of organicism as a paradigm distinct
from both mechanism and vitalism. To conclude, we will survey
Harrison, Needham, and Weiss from an enriched philosophical and
historical vantage point.

Mastermann insists that the artefact component of paradigms is
useful precisely because it is crude. "If a paradigm has got to have the
property of concreteness, or 'crudeness,' this means that it must be,
literally, a model; or, literally, a picture; or, literally, an analogy-
drawing sequence of word-uses in natural language; or some combination of these" (1970, p. 79). The concrete nature of models,
metaphors, and artefacts, is essential to science because it limits the
implications of any particular abstract system. A set of mathematical
relations and operational terms of a well-developed science can be
dangerously overextended. The crudeness of a paradigm picture both
stimulates and bounds the imagination, giving direction to the power
of abstract expression and linking the contributions of *images* private
to a particular scientist, *words* that aim to communicate insight and
theories that formalize tested common understanding. The concrete
artefact, an actual object constructed by an investigator to explore
his insights, is a puzzle-solving device. It is possible to tell when a
solution works. The use of real objects in the solution of DNA's structure
is a striking example of the power of artefacts in biology even if they
have possibly outlived their relevance in modern physics. A picture,
metaphor, or model developed in words is like an object; it can be
pushed too far in exploring something else. An overextended metaphor
ruins a poem; an analogy in biology runs aground when wrongly
applied. The misapplication by eighteenth-century iatromechanists of
the popular literal machine analogy to the physiology of the organism
is a notorious example; the fruitfulness of the analogy of the organism
as an energy conversion machine in the nineteenth century shows the
positive potential.

With Harrison, Needham, and Weiss the crude dimension of paradigms is strikingly evident. Several images were repeatedly developed

by these workers and their associates: liquid crystal (all three biologists, to illuminate protoplasmic structure), railway switchyard (Needham, to suggest successive determinations in embryogenesis), topographical models (Waddington and Needham, to propose a system of probabilities and progressive limitations in developmental pathways), and replicating subpatterns (Weiss, to probe cell structure and hierarchical organization). Harrison kept a room full of artefacts to help him think out the aspects of organismic symmetries and asymmetries. Needham's imagination was aroused by Harrison's and Bernal's strongly visual and manual working out of ideas. All these gross analogies grew out of organismic biases; they were attempts to visualize wholeness so the abstraction could be translated into common, scientific, systematic understanding. All these analogies contributed to puzzle-solving activities, and all could certainly be pressed too far. Harrison's early suspicion that the tetrahedral carbon atom might be the immediate basis of molecular arrangement and thus of limb symmetry proved too simple; the metaphor could not carry the weight. The more complicated image of liquid crystals was at various times both an analogy and a picture taken literally. From both points of view, the crude aspects of the organismic paradigm guided research and allowed communication among diverse, scattered persons. In the opinion of this author the paradigm notion in its clothing of analogy and metaphor is of great use in tracing the growth of ideas in developmental biology. The specific switches of metaphor illuminate deep underlying changes of perspective on the nature of the organism.

The sociological paradigm highlights the role of distinct communities. Kuhn stresses that different paradigm communities talk past one another because they do not use the same words to mean the same thing. For example, perhaps the concept of structure was not the same for an organicist such as Harrison and a mechanist such as Weismann. If the paradigm notion is to be useful in studying the growth of biology, clearly demarcated groups sharing ideas, images, tools, and concrete problems should be evident. Kuhn feels that a science matures when the constant unresolvable philosophical debates of a preparadigm phase give way to a dominant guiding framework, a true paradigm. Persons embracing different paradigms, possible for sciences offering more than one functioning perspective or during a period of revolutionary change of perspective, should at least have trouble talking with one another. Kuhn believes that his differences of opinion with

Karl Popper over the nature of progress in science illustrate the incommensurable dimensions of different paradigms. Is this understanding of paradigm communities helpful in analyzing the development of cell biology and embryology represented by Harrison, Needham, and Weiss? Does there have to be a single or even a dominant paradigm in order for a field to be scientific? How closely knit must paradigm groups be? Answers to these questions are essential if we are to decide if a new paradigm appeared in this century.

Paul Feyerabend criticizes Kuhn's suggestion of noncommunicating paradigm groups for artificially obscuring the elements of fruitful conflict and interchange of views among individuals and groups in science. He feels there is less a succession of crises, suggested by the idea of paradigm revolution and closed groups, than a constant interplay; tenaciously held views do not preclude comprehension and conflict. Feyerabend fears that Kuhn is proposing that progress in knowledge is achieved at the price of diversity and communication among those who differ (1970). However, the idea of paradigm communities need not be so stringent. Partial blocks in communication do appear to characterize those working from different perspectives, but Kuhn's idea might be more useful in exploring the positive function of communities than in drawing tight boundaries between groups and in deciding which perspective is dominant. Especially in tracing the subtleties of mechanism and vitalism, and of organicism and neo-mechanism or reductionism, the more relaxed definition of paradigm community is necessary. Rarely does a person fit into one group to the exclusion of others. Even the Theoretical Biology Club, the exemplary paradigm community suggested by this book, did not tightly define the allegiances of its members, but the TBC did help reveal similarities in perception and interpretation of problems. It did draw persons from many areas into a coherent, exciting, if plastic, group. In a later section of this chapter the question of paradigm communities will come up again. It will be necessary to decide if Harrison, Needham, and Weiss truly shared a common paradigm, or if the differences among them might make the suggestion of a unifying organicism misleading. At that time it will be important to remember the caution that the community dimension of paradigms need not be taken to the extreme to be revealing.

Closely associated with evaluating the relevance of the sociological paradigm is a consideration of the suggested revolutionary aspect of

paradigms. Is there really a difference between normal science within
a functioning paradigm and periods of crisis and revolution? How can
one tell if there has been a change in paradigm? For the historian,
after a while the continuities in societies before and after supposed
revolutions loom much larger than the discontinuities. Revolutions
look ultimately conservative. Granted that there are difficult times of
strain and that ideas are discarded in favor of others, does it really
help to see the changes in science through the glasses of revolution?
Change is a matter of degree. If discontinuities are frequent, the idea
of revolution could become trivial. Perhaps the microstructure of
revolution is normal science. Then what becomes of the guiding idea
of paradigms? (Toulmin 1970). Toulmin draws the analogy of the
debate between catastrophism and uniformitarianism or evolutionism
in geology. In the end geologists had to look at actual mechanisms of
change and found neither idea adequate. Toulmin contends that
change in ideas could be better visualized through the spectacles of
constant variation and selection of the fittest, rather than of saltatory
evolution. But Toulmin's criticism does not demonstrate that opposing
ideas in geology did not define the controversy and suggest precisely
how to look for actual mechanisms of change. Again, in retrospect,
revolutions always appear conservative. Kuhn explains this fact by
showing how the survivors of revolutionary paradigm change write
history as if it were simple and progressive. Past opponents must be
either forerunners of the present truth or practitioners of something
short of real science. Current opponents must be wrong. In a later
portion of this chapter a critical eye will be cast on Harrison, Needham,
and Weiss in relation to the proposed revolutionary change in paradigm from the polarities of mechanism and vitalism to the new frame
of organicism. Again, we must ask to what extent the three shared the
same paradigm and participated in the same revolution in developmental biology, if indeed revolution be a useful word here. Perhaps a
microanalysis of the context in which they worked would dissolve the
apparent discontinuities traced in the earlier chapters of this book.

I have included Mastermann's category of metaparadigm in this
volume's consideration of paradigm revolution in order to stress the
multiple philosophical and extraexperimental elements of paradigms.
If there has been a revolutionary paradigm change, organicism must
be substantively different from either mechanism or vitalism. But one
cannot assume this distinction. Perhaps the strains of organicism in

Harrison, Needham, and Weiss are variations on old themes, not contributions to a new score. Kuhn's model fails to illuminate the work of these three biologists, especially considered together, if a case cannot be made for radical, discontinuous change in understanding of the nature of the organism in the period under study. So before we turn to a careful comparison and contrast of Harrison, Needham, and Weiss according to the paradigm categories of model, community, and revolution, it is essential to probe more deeply into the relation of organicism to other interpretations of the organism and of the science of biology.

Hilde Hein argues that organicism must be considered a modern variant of vitalism and that the old categories of mechanism and vitalism are still very much relevant to the contemporary biological scene. She emphasizes paradigm distinctions in biology but rejects the notion that the parameters of paradigms have changed markedly in this century (1971). She claims that contemporary mechanists and vitalists oppose each other mainly by citing an outdated form of the other's perspective and showing that it is untenable. But the adherents to the two perspectives remain divided by fundamental intellectual choices that will never submit to empirical decision, although one may cite reasons for preferring one approach over the other. In her chapter on vitalism she recognizes several forms: vital force theories, entelechies, theories of emergent evolution, and organicism. The last two are the modern manifestations of an ancient insistence on using more than one set of principles for explaining nature. In other words vitalists are dualists before they enter a laboratory; they exist in a plural world comprehended in plural terms never to be collapsed into one another. For reasons that escape pure experimental observation, the distinction between living and nonliving must not be allowed to blur. The changing faces of mechanism—from Greek atomism and the search for the unchanging one underlying all apparent change through theories using machine metaphors evolving from clock to hydraulic device and heat engine to computer—are but masks on a basic conviction that the world must yield to a single set of explanatory principles rigorously and commonly interpreted. Historically, each vitalist challenge has been countered by a more refined mechanism, only to reappear in new guise. Vital substance theories such as that of John Needham (1713–1781) were undermined by advances in chemical synthesis and organic analysis. Vital energy theories were overthrown definitively by the demonstration that organisms must submit to the first law of thermodynamics. The most recent vitalists, Hein maintains, no longer argue for special vital matter or energy but for special biological laws not reducible to those of physics and chemistry. Metaphysical vitalism has been abandoned for epistemological assertions.

In chapter 2 it was stressed that all twentieth-century organicists have resisted reduction of biology to physics and chemistry. Organicism transcended the dichotomies of mechanism and vitalism but maintained a special place for the whole organism by proposing unique biological laws of integration and organization. Remember that Joseph Woodger in *Biological Principles*, in a statement later adopted by Needham, defined vitalism as any doctrine that posited some entity or force in organisms in addition to the chemical elements plus organizing relations. His organicism rested solely on a belief in independent biological principles of organization. What do such assertions imply and can they be maintained? If autonomy of a science means anything, it is that the laws and terms of one science cannot without loss be translated into the terms of another. "In a complete reduction, the laws of the reduced science may, with the help of certain 'rules of transformation' be deduced from the laws and principles of the reducing science." In itself, the issue of reductionism does not prejudice the question of whether the language of translation comes from disciplines dealing with objects of supposedly greater or lesser complexity. Indeed, a few thinkers have maintained that the laws of physics and chemistry will eventually be "reduced" to those of biology. C. F. A. Pantin, discussed in chapter 1, approaches a variation of that position. Thus, autonomy of a science means logical independence: The same event or object could be explained from two or more points of view, and the descriptions would be incommensurable and complementary rather than logically redundant. Note that the claimed "autonomy of the laws [of an independent science] is with respect to one another, not to events" (Hein 1970, pp. 170, 174). No one claims that, at present, any portion of biology has been fully reduced to physics, although certain areas in molecular genetics might come close. Further, it is not claimed even that it would be profitable to attempt to reduce entirely all aspects of what is commonly called biology to any other science, much less to quantum mechanics, for example. The most ardent reductionists allow for the heuristic function of specifically biological laws and investigations (Beckner 1967).

One simple reason that full reduction is not currently possible, even if it were desirable, is that biology is not fully axiomatized. Clearly, complete logical reduction implies that both sets of principles have that property. J. H. Woodger, a very important organicist, has spent his life working on the axiomatization of a small segment of Mendelian genetics. C. H. Waddington, in his series *Towards a Theoretical Biology*, has also attempted to find biological laws that lend themselves to a high degree of logical and mathematical formalization. Both these workers would deny that biology's attainment of this particular form of scientific maturity would result in ultimate reduction to the laws of physics. Each would assert that biological principles will show themselves to be unique. For them the autonomy of biology will reside in biology's own mature statement of abstract, systematized laws. For others axiomatization would be a prelude to more complete reduction.

However, the significant aspect of these debates is the common assumption that the only remaining issue is epistemological, not metaphysical. But traditional mechanists and vitalists argued as much over the existence of vital substance or energy as over the status of generalizations. In addition to metaphysical and epistemological issues, the old debate also involved specific methodological disagreements, for example whether analysis applied to biology was more than thanatology. Needham spent some time in his *Order and Life* defending analysis in his science; he believed that his position differentiated him from various vitalists. Paul Weiss leaned more to traditional vitalism in his polemics over the origin of life. For him it would be *practically* impossible to synthesize living organisms in the laboratory; the division of living and nonliving is, at that point, fundamental. Also, he held that unique laws are required to understand the organization of the living world. Few contemporary organicists would reassert with Weiss the ultimate practical division of organic and inorganic. Nevertheless, argument over the logical status of generalizations raises great and persistent passions.

The question of the existence of a new paradigm may now be rephrased. Is the vitalism–mechanism debate equivalent to the contemporary organicism–reductionism (or neomechanism) controversy? The very juxtaposition in terminology of reductionism, a word relating clearly to epistemology, with neomechanism, an expression relating naturally to positions on substance or metaphysics, would argue the appropriateness of the equation. Hein would then be justified in

treating organicism as a form of vitalism. But several important objections must be raised. Key changes in the meanings of words might
give sufficient ground for asserting the existence of substantially new
paradigms competing for biologists' allegiance.

First, why has the debate over vital substance or energy evaporated?
Beyond the obvious significance of advances in sophistication of observation and experiment, such that it is ridiculous to maintain that
organisms contain unique matter, the meaning of the word *substance*
has changed for both biology and phycis. It is common knowledge
that the matter of modern physics posits organization and motion at
its core. There are no more inert ultimate units pushed around from
the outside. Matter and energy are ultimately equivalent. In other
sections of this book the importance of these changes, as evidenced by
Whitehead's popular exposition of 1925, has been outlined. In addition to a liberated concept of matter, modern physical science (and
other fields commonly seen as contemporary mechanistic triumphs)
employ an expanded version of the machine metaphor. The computer
that is capable of learning, has a memory, and can even reproduce is
a far cry from a clock, pump, or steam engine. In fact the metaphor
of the computer has been found very useful by doctrinaire organicists
such as Weiss. A convergence of metaphor signals fundamental alteration in paradigm assumptions. Third, modern mechanism even
has adapted to notions of evolution and apparent directiveness. The
synthetic theory of evolution and doctrines of the development of
matter in the cosmos testify to this startling dimension of so-called
mechanism. Obviously, the use of the term *mechanism* is difficult, if not
impossible, if one is historically sensitive to its various meanings. The
expression *reductionism* conveys much better the basic assertions of contemporary thinkers. It is hard to defend the equivalence of traditional
mechanism and modern reductionism without losing the flavor of the
old debate and missing the revolutionary significance of the modern
transformation.

It is equally difficult to insist on the identity of vitalism and organicism. Whereas the earlier notions of physics made the task of
biology—the explanation of form, regulation, and organization—virtually impossible without imputing some spiritual force or extraordinary matter, contemporary fundamental ideas about the nature of the
cosmos allow biologists great hope in their own field. Organization
could become a problem rather than an evasion through an excessively
narrow world view. Woodger maintained that the early years of this

century would be remembered as the time in which scientists first sought seriously an adequate theory of organisms. Needham launched into polemics at the least hint that organization was not soluble. Organicists of every hue have averred that it is not appropriate to look outside science for an understanding of organisms. Vitalists were, at the very least, not so sure. Therefore, although both vitalists and organicists share a devotion to the idea of wholeness and a rejection of mechanistic physics and chemistry as adequate to the solution of biological problems, they diverge on a very critical issue. Organicists declare that it will be possible to state positive, unambiguous, empirically grounded laws for all aspects of the behavior of organisms. Form and organization are not mysteries, but challenges.

Nevertheless, Hein is correct in insisting strongly that essential elements of a very traditional dispute are retained in contemporary biology. It is wholly misleading to assert the dominance of a single perspective on many issues, such as identification of the most important problems for study. In the early days of explicit organicism, Ritter railed against the tyranny of Mendelian genetics at the expense of whole organism biology. Morgan's digression was getting out of hand. Today also, the place granted to genetics is a good indicator of the overall allegiance of a worker. In general, organicists are suspicious of the excitement surrounding molecular biology. For example, in his film *Assault on Life*, Barry Commoner argues that the only key to life is life. He is emotionally emphasizing the basic commitment to the organism as the fundamental unit of biological study and the legitimacy of seeking "autonomous" biological laws.

At this point it is necessary to qualify the position that only an epistemological disagreement separates organicists and reductionists. Why should it make a difference if logical reduction were theoretically possible, as long as everyone grants everyone else the untrammeled right to pursue problems of interest without insisting on actual reductions? In a very provocative little book Michael Simon persuasively argues that persons choose different styles of investigation and explanation for specifically human purposes, not because of any particular properties of the nonhuman world (1971). Hein holds the same opinion: events and objects are not at stake, only the way we choose to express ourselves. But the issue is not so simple. Organicists tend not to agree with Kant. This fact puts them in the embarrassing position of naked philosophical realism.

Woodger put it boldly, if ungracefully, when he wrote to Needham that his early neomechanism was wrong because "knowledge requires to have a structure which reflects the structure of fact and to be adequate, its structure has to be of the same degree of manifoldness as that of fact."[1] Needham felt in this period of his development that he must proceed *as if* the world could be rigorously explained by mechanistic, or better, reductionistic science. Curiously, he held this opinion because he thought it protected the equally absolute rights of other kinds of understanding and experience (e.g., religion) in their proper spheres. Tight methodological monism in science was the price for allowing multiple kinds of experience in life. Like a good scientific reductionist, he made no explicit metaphysical claims; mechanism and materialism do not imply each other. From his later organismic vantage point, Needham no longer believed that such high walls had to be erected between science and religion. Ironically, the assertion of the autonomy of biological laws permitted him to structure the world into a unified hierarchy. His evolutionary succession of types of organization from atoms to world commonwealths replaced his earlier separate but equal spheres. For Needham each level led to studies with a limited but critical autonomy because no level or field of inquiry was ultimately the only foundation stone.

Paul Weiss went even further than Needham. He reasoned that man's imaginative and cognitive powers derived from his sharing common patterns of organization with the rest of nature. Knowledge reflected the patterns of the world because it too is built on the same fundamental structure. He would deny that reductionism versus organicism comes to nothing more than an argument about how to classify and manipulate generalizations. One adopts a particular form of study and judges its importance according to one's assumptions about the nature of things. It is useful to recall Hein's key point: The barrier separating organicists and reductionists will not be breached by empirical study, because in the end people believe different things about the structure of the world. Emotional, psychological, and political elements deeply condition the starting points.

Therefore, the position of this study is that there exists a basic difference between vitalists and organicists that rests on a switch from metaphysical to epistemological debate. But embedded in the epistemo-

1. Correspondence from Woodger to Needham, February 1, 1930. See pp. 110–11*n* of this study.

logical claims remains a root belief that science can reveal nature. Biology must be autonomous because organisms are somehow different and unique, even if no clear explanation is given to show precisely how one can know that. Reductionists allow organicists to proceed *as if* their field were logically and really independent, but at heart they believe that the truth is elsewhere. In like manner, organicists allow reductionists to proceed *as if* the world were single and simple but know that wisdom eludes them. Each approach encounters its own limitations. Historically, both vitalists and organicists have trouble accounting for the unity of physical nature, for the bond between organic and inorganic; but organicists at least are well able to bridge the gulf between mind and body. Mechanists see no problem in the unity of living and nonliving but often have failed badly in inquiries requiring the union of mind and body. Reductionists pretend to make no claims about reality but by default assert that nothing is more than useful and methodological. The world should be approached in univocal terms because there is no plural, polyvocal nature. Or at least we cannot know it. In summary then, it is possible to maintain that there is a crucial discontinuity between vitalism–mechanism and organicism–reductionism. There has been a paradigm change, but a basic duality is preserved around a very important, if unresolvable, issue: Is the world one or many? Is knowledge literal and single or metaphoric and plural?

It is time to return to a specific analysis of our three principal figures: Harrison, Needham, and Weiss. Some have asserted that organicists felt they were doing something new, something beyond the dead ends encountered by mechanism and vitalism. However, it is not evident how far they were right on a day-to-day basis. In addition it is not apparent yet whether organicism as we have encountered it in this book is a single, coherent perspective or an array of unrelated positions. A final picture of the organismic paradigm requires some additional brushwork.

Obviously the study of wholeness in development did not begin with Ross Harrison. His work grew naturally out of the concerns of developmental biology in the late nineteenth century. Roux had set the stage and asked the principal questions about self versus dependent differentiation. Investigation "on the biological level" was well underway with no great splits between organicist and reductionist. Moreover, attention was focused on the structure of protoplasm and on ways to link structure and function, to reveal process through clear perception of structure. Even the extreme preformationist theory of Weismann with its structured idioplasm contains a sense of hierarchical organization of protoplasm and the close tie of form to process. But the structure of chromatin, the key component of the cell, was rigidly fixed and transmitted from generation to generation without change. Harrison's conception of dynamic molecular structure was radically different. Further, Weismann went way beyond what he could assert from observation about mitosis and qualitative division. Many others had also speculated about complex molecules that might explain cellular processes; Spencer had his physiological units, Darwin his gemmules, De Vries his pangens, Nageli his micelles, Hertwig his idioblasts, and Verworn his biogens (Wilson 1896, p. 22).

With his usual acumen E. B. Wilson explained how positions such as his own and that of Harrison differed from the preformationist camp's search for simple, rigid subunits that would explain the workings of the organism machine. Complexity and wholeness are the key ideas.

> The truth is that an explanation of development is at present beyond our reach. The controversy between preformation and epigenesis has now arrived at a stage where it has little meaning apart from the general problem of physical causality. ... The second question, regarding the historical origin of the idioplasm, brings us to the side of the evolutionists. ... Whatever position we take on this question, the same difficulty is encountered; namely the origin of that co-ordinated fitness, that power of active adjustment between internal and external relations. ... The nature and origin of this power is the fundamental problem of biology. [pp. 328–29]

Wilson reaffirmed his belief that organic nature is a finely graded series from lower to higher forms and that all differences in complexity have a natural origin. But having considered all qualifications, he concluded that "the study of the cell has on the whole seemed to widen rather than narrow the enormous gap that separates even the lowest forms of life from the inorganic world" (p. 330).

Wilson did not deny that eventually the ultimate questions of biology would be scientifically answered. He only insisted that the problems were enormously complex and that the simpler solutions based on a machine metaphor were inadequate. Reserving final judgment, he saw his field alive with exciting empirical investigations into the cell in heredity and development. His own bias was undogmatically organismic; he constantly stressed the need to know how the cell or any part functioned in the whole, how coordination occurs. The division between organic and inorganic was a practical fact, if not a final one. His work represents one of the first systematic attempts to give concrete content to the problem of biological organization. Harrison fits in that tradition. He did not begin a radically new school by building a new paradigm in contrast to a well-defined mechanistic opposition. Rather, he belongs to the first generation that made explicit experimental investigations into developmental processes of coordination. As Ritter noted, one of the important roots of contemporary organicism is to be found in the American school of embryology, but these early organicists did not differentiate themselves markedly from contemporary mechanists. Instead they shared problems and approaches, differing more in stress and interpretation than in dogma.

As Harrison began his work on limb symmetry, he moved more deeply into the organismic paradigm with its natural metaphors and community associations. He was led to contemplate the molecular basis of symmetry and to adopt the liquid crystal image with its implication of dynamic structure. He was excited by Needham's Terry Lectures and sought out Astbury to collaborate on electron microscope work. Finally, in his own Silliman Lectures he formulated his theory of the organism and development. We have seen in the second section of chapter 3 precisely how that theory was based on an organismic paradigm (see pp. 94–100 above). We have also traced the connection of Harrison's views on the matter with Needham's.

Harrison assiduously avoided polemics and philosophical extremes. He was a typical nineteenth-century agnostic liberal (who nonetheless voted for Eugene Debs for president because of his imprisonment for political reasons). His bent was toward careful experimental investigation of large problems. His syntheses and overall directions were always definitely linked to work in the laboratory. Such a person is ill suited to participate in the more dogmatic aspects of paradigm building. His organicism is not identical to that of Needham and Weiss, both because Harrison's problems emerged from different earlier traditions (developmental mechanics instead of biochemistry or animal behavior and engineering) and because he would not commit himself on an ultimate position on the autonomy of biological laws. According to Hein's criterion, Harrison was in the end a qualified reductionist: he tended to believe that a single set of principles would result from science. In the meantime he did not press this conviction. He reasoned that it would be more rewarding to examine the possibilities of investigation on every level of organization. But according to more relaxed criteria, Harrison was a qualified organicist. His choice of problems, his style of interpretation, his favorite metaphors, his intellectual fraternity—all were appropriate to the organismic paradigm. He rejected the over-simplifications of machine-model interpretations of development. His own work, a major contribution to field theory, underlies the best current work on systematic and dynamic patterns. Kuhn's notion is partially useful in understanding Harrison's significance, but the idea must not be overextended.

For Joseph Needham, Kuhn's model is much more helpful, perhaps because Needham was so much more given to explaining the changes in his ideas. He was led into organicism as much or more by philosophical and political opinions as by the requirements of his experimental material. There is a definite break in Needham's thought and work. He associated with a different group, namely, the Theoretical Biology Club. His images changed from automotive gear shifts to fields, or-ganizers, and liquid crystals. Drawing on the strong visual thinking of Bernal, Waddington, and Harrison and on the philosophical per-spectives of Woodger, Engels, and Whitehead, Needham rerouted his whole mode of thought and experiment. He felt he was participating in a major change in biological framework. Indeed, he felt that his organicism was quite different from that of Haldane and Russell, so much so that he classified the latter two as vitalists. From a greater distance this split is less defensible. Needham had a tendency to begin with the solution to a problem and to develop language and experi-ments suitable to his conviction. Use of the terminology of individuation and evocation is an example. Harrison found these terms a bit funny, if not mysterious, but in the end, Harrison and Needham spoke of the organism in very similar terms. They shared language, images, and experimental concerns.

Needham's intense belief in social progress conditioned his percep-tion of the nature of the division between organic and inorganic. He regarded biology as an autonomous science—its generalizations would remain logically independent from those of physics and chemistry.

However, there existed a continuous, graded series of levels of complexity. He did not separate the levels of the cosmic hierarchy to the same extent that Weiss did but perhaps more than Harrison would permit. According to Hein's criterion, Needham must be classified an unqualified organicist. Further, the notion of paradigm revolution illuminates his intellectual development.

The paradigm model is useful in looking at Paul Weiss as well. He interpreted his own work in revolutionary terms, early in relation to the framework of Jacques Loeb and later in relation to the reductionist camp. According to all three criteria of metaphor and language, community association, and revolution, Weiss worked within a definable organismic paradigm. But he is separate from the organicism of Harrison and Needham; he is more extreme. Over the problem of continuity between organic and inorganic, the origin of life, Weiss separated himself. From Hein's perspective he should be called a vitalist. It is interesting to compare Weiss's article in *Beyond Reductionism* with Waddington's work in the series *Towards a Theoretical Biology*. If both individual contributions, and indeed the overall direction represented by both volumes, are forms of organicism, they are critically different as well. The participants in the Alpbach group, within which Waddington held himself apart, leaned toward vitalism on two issues: the origin of life (the unabridgeable split between living and nonliving) and evolution (the role of inheritance of acquired characteristics and a mysterious kind of directive force).[2] Both Waddington and Weiss tend to reason mathematically more than Harrison or Needham, but they use mathematical tools for different ends. Clearly, the division between organicism and reductionism or between variants of organicism does not lie in the presence or absence of mathematics.

Let us return to the general questions of this chapter. Is Kuhn's model useful in this area of biology? If so, has a new paradigm arisen? And do Harrison, Needham, and Weiss really share the same paradigm? In his reply to his critics in *Criticism and the Growth of Knowledge*, Kuhn argues that distinct paradigm groups should show partial incomprehension of one anothers' views and talk past one another on crucial issues. This property characterizes the mechanism–vitalism debate as well as the controversy between organicists and reductionists. Moreover, it has already been established that there are good grounds

2. For a good discussion of these matters, see Joravsky 1972, pp. 23–25.

for separating the contemporary dispute from the traditional one. The positive evidence for a revolutionary change in Harrison's, Needham's, and Weiss's perspectives comes from restructuring of group commitments, change of language and metaphor, and reorientation of experimental concerns and interpretations. For example, even before Harrison had finished his research on the limb field, and thus before his organicism was fully explicit, he identified a crisis in anatomy by contending that animal structure should be studied as formative process. Negative evidence, strongest for Harrison, arises from the continuity of work on basic questions, such as the relation of cell to organism, among so-called mechanists such as Weismann and organicists such as Wilson or Harrison. Furthermore, Kuhn's idea that establishment of a new dominant paradigm should result in a period of progress and normal science and in the death of previous polemics does not apply. Organicists, a minority group in terms of overt allegiance to the framework, continue to engage in polemics, often in vague terms that are hard to relate to actual experimental issues. Most biologists would admit that even today no adequate theory of the organism exists, from whatever perspective. In that sense, biology has not reached the paradigm phase of development. But however mature the science according to the standards of theoretical physics, a great deal of theory and practice exists for which the paradigm model is enlightening.

Harrison, Needham, and Weiss differ in their spontaneous use of visual imagery, but they borrow from common sources so that in the end they are quite similar. They vary also in their perception of belonging to distinct paradigm communities and in their final positions on the continuity of living and nonliving. Nevertheless, they are closely related in their insistence that form is the central focus of biology, in their choice of experimental problems appropriate to organicist interpretations, in their lack of conviction that genetics is the key to biology, and in their use of revealing metaphors such as liquid crystal and field. Seeing problem sets to be like one another is a basic quality of a shared paradigm. They are inclined to agree in their interpretations of hierarchical organization in cell structure, organismic symmetry, and overlapping fields.

It is possible to argue that the organicism of Harrison and Needham, and often that of Weiss, is really a variant of contemporary neomechanism or reductionism rather than either a variant of vitalism or an entirely new paradigm. But this position is unhelpful. Let us look at a partial list of metaphors, objects, and problems that are relevant from three different perspectives. The traditional mechanist sees similarities between the organism and actual machines such as the steam engine, hydraulic pump, or a system of levers and pulleys. The neomechanist builds a similarity set from codes, the molecular basis of genes, language, computers, and the organism. In this context the word *mechanist* is used only to indicate a particular tendency to single out problems and metaphors, not to indicate a philosophical dogma. The organicist tends to see similarities in the structure of molecular populations, the cell, the whole organism, and the ecosystem. System laws would apply at each level. Concrete analogies are drawn from models, gestalt phenomena, fields, liquid crystals, and also computers. These lists suggest that persons holding one of the three perspectives would be inclined to work on different experimental problems and to interpret the results in different language. There is significant overlap among all three categories; for example, both organicists and neomechanists are interested in cytoplasmic structure and in computers. Recognizing paradigm commitment is similar to the problem of recognizing biological species. It is inappropriate to rely on a single type but crucial to cluster objects into similarity sets. Thus we return to the illative sense described in chapter 2, which allows a person to recognize what is like and unlike. For Harrison the limb field is like a liquid crystal and unlike a jigsaw puzzle. For Needham the embryo is like history interpreted from a Marxist viewpoint and unlike an automobile with gear shifts. For Weiss butterfly behavior is like a random search and self-correcting device and unlike a deterministic stimulus–response machine. Such a catalog could be continued indefinitely, but the basic point is that organicists, even granting their internal differences, share central perceptions on the level of images and language. These perceptions underlie their philosophical and explicit verbal commitments. We are indebted to Kuhn for stressing the extralogical dimensions of scientific investigation. Using the paradigm model as a tool, we are able to see some of the role of the imagination and emotion in theory building.

But most important, we can discern the fundamental differences between organicist and reductionist. From their emotional, psychological, and linguistic preferences, we see that organicists continually return to a modified philosophical realism. The debate over the status of laws becomes a debate over the nature of form. Organicists reject the reductionistic approach primarily because they refuse to see the world in single terms. They share a root faith that the task of the scientist is not merely to order and test our own generalizations. Experimentally grounded organicism has aimed at constructing a reformed realism that would contribute to the great poet–scientist's goal "to restore to the intellect its old privilege of taking a direct view of nature" (Goethe 1952, p. 238). Ross Harrison's deep admiration for Goethe was seminal and prophetic.

References

Abercrombie, M.
 1961. Ross Granville Harrison. Proceedings of the Royal Society. *Biograph. Mem. Fellows Roy. Soc.* 7: 110–26.
Arber, Agnes
 1954. *The Mind and the Eye*. London: Cambridge University Press.
Astbury, W. T.
 1939. X-ray studies of the structure of compounds of biological interest. *Ann. Rev. Biochem.* 8: 113–32.
Baitsell, George A.
 1940. A modern concept of the cell as a structural unit. *Am. Nat.* 74:5–24.
Baltzer, Fritz
 1967. *Theodor Boveri: Life and Work of a Great Biologist*. Berkeley and Los Angeles: University of California Press.
Beckner, Morton O.
 1967. Organismic biology. In *The Encyclopedia of Philosophy*, ed. Paul Edwards. Vol. 5. New York: Macmillan Co. and The Free Press.
Bertalanffy, Ludwig von
 1933. *Modern Theories of Development*, trans. J. H. Woodger. London: Oxford University Press (Berlin: Borntraeger, 1928).
 1952. *Problems of Life*. London: Watts and Company.
Black, Max
 1962. *Models and Metaphors*. Ithaca, N.Y.: Cornell University Press.
Boell, E. J.; Needham, J.; and Rogers, Veronica
 1939. Morphogenesis and metabolism: Studies with the Cartesian diver and ultramicromanometer. I. Anaerobic glycolysis of the regions of the amphibian gastrula. *Proc. Roy. Soc. London, Ser. B* 127: 322–56.
Boell, E. J., and Needham, J.
 1939a. II. Effect of dinitro-o-cresol on the anaerobic glycolysis of the regions of the amphibian gastrula. *Proc. Roy. Soc. London, Ser. B* 127: 356–62.
 1939b. III. Respiratory rate of the regions of the amphibian gastrula. *Proc. Roy. Soc. London, Ser. B* 127: 363–73.
Boell, E. J.; Koch, Henri; and Needham, J.
 1939. IV. Respiratory quotient of the regions of the amphibian gastrula. *Proc. Roy. Soc. London, Ser. B* 127: 374–87.

Boveri, Theodor
    1901. Ueber die Polarität des Seeigeleies. *Verhandl. Phys.-Med. Ges. Würzburg, NF* 34: 145–76.
Bridgman, P. W.
    1927. *Logic of Modern Physics.* New York: Macmillan.
Brooke, John H.
    1968. Wöhler's urea and its vital force?—A verdict from the chemists. *Ambix* 15: 84–113.
Bruni, A., and Racker, E.
    1968. Resolution and reconstitution of the mitochondrial electron transport system. *J. Biol Chem.* 243: 962–71.
Campbell, N. R.
    1920. *Physics, the Elements.* London: Cambridge University Press.
Child, C. M.
    1941. *Patterns and Problems of Development.* Chicago: Chicago University Press.
Churchill, Frederick B.
    1968. August Weismann and a break from tradition. *J. Hist. Biol* 1: 91–112.
Coleman, William
    1971. *Biology in the Nineteenth Century.* New York: John Wiley and Sons.
Crick, Francis
    1966. *Of Molecules and Men.* Seattle: University of Washington Press.
Descartes, René
    1955. *Philosophical Works of Descartes*, trans. E. S. Haklane and G. Ross. New York: Dover Publications.
Driesch, Hans
    1894. *Analytische Theorie der organischen Entwicklung.* Leipzig: Wilhelm Engelmann.
    1929. *The Science and Philosophy of the Organism*, 2nd ed. London: Black.
Duhem, Pierre
    1914. *La théorie physique.* Paris: M. Rivière.
Einstein, Albert, and Infeld, I.
    1938. *The Evolution of Physics.* London: Cambridge University Press.
Engels, Frederick
    1940. *Dialectics of Nature.* Clemens Dutt (trans.). New York: International Publishers.
Feyerabend, Paul
    1970. Consolations for the specialist. In *Criticism and the Growth of Knowledge.* London: Cambridge University Press.
Foucault, Michel
    1970. *The Order of Things.* New York: Pantheon Books.

Galaty, David H.
  1974. The philosophical basis of mid-nineteenth century reductionism. *J. Hist. Med. Allied Sci.* 29: 295–316.
Galbiani, G., ed.
  1967. *Reflections on Biological Research.* St Louis: W. H. Green.
Gilbert, W., and Miller-Hill, B.
  1966. The isolation of the lac repressor. *Proc. Nat. Acad. Sci.* 56: 1891–98.
Goethe, Johann Ludwig von
  1952. Analysis and synthesis. In *Goethe's Botannical Writings*, trans. Berthe Mueller. Honolulu: University of Hawaii Press.
Goodfield, June
  1969. Theories and hypotheses in biology. In *Boston Studies in the Philosophy of Science*, V, ed. Robert Cohen. Pp. 421–49. Dordrecht: D. Reidel.
Grew, Nehemiah
  1965. *The Anatomy of Plants. The Sources of Science*, no. 11. ed. Harry Woolf. New York: Johnson Reprint.
Gurwitsch, A.
  1922. Über den Begriff des embryonalen Feldes. *Arch. Entwicklungsmech. Organ.* 51: 383–415.
  1927. Weiterbildung und Verallgemeinerung des Feldbegriffes. *Arch. Entwicklungsmech. Organ.* 112: 433–54.
Haldane, J. S.
  1917. *Organism and Environment.* New Haven: Yale University Press.
  1931. *Philosophical Basis of Biology.* London: Hodden and Stoughton.
Haldane, J. S., and Priestley, J. H.
  1935. *Respiration.* Oxford: Clarendon Press.
Hamburger, V.
  1969. Hans Spemann and the organizer concept. *Experientia* 25: 1121–25.
Hardy, W. B.
  1899. On the structure of cell-protoplasm: The structure produced in a cell by fixative and post-mortem change, the structure of colloid matter, and the mechanism of setting and coagulation. *J. Physiol.* 24: 288.
Harrison, Ross G.
  1894. The development of the fins of teleosts. *Johns Hopkins Univ. Circ.* 13: 59–61.
  1898. The growth and regeneration of the tail of the frog larva. Studied with the aid of Born's method of grafting. *Arch. Entwicklungsmech. Organ.* 7: 430–85.
  1901. The histogenesis of the peripheral nervous system in *Salmo salar. Biol. Bull.* 2: 352–53.
  1903a. On the differentiation of muscular tissue when removed from the influence of the nervous system. *Am. J. Anat.* 2: iv–v.

1903*b*. Experimentelle Untersuchungen über die Entwicklung der Sinnesorgane der Seitenlinie bei den Amphibien. *Arch. Mikroskop. Anat.* 63: 35–149.

1904*a*. An experimental study of the relation of the nervous system to the developing musculature in the embryo of the frog. *Am. J. Anat.* 3: 197–220.

1904*b*. Neue Versuche und Beobachtungen über die Entwicklung der peripheren Nerven der Wirbeltiere. Sitzungsberichte d. Niederrhein. *Gesellschaft für Natur- und Heilkunde. Bonn. Jahrg.* pp. 1–7.

1906. Further experiments on the development of peripheral nerves. *Am. J. Anat.* 5: 121–31.

1907*a*. Experiments in transplanting limbs and their bearing on the problems of the development of nerves. (Abstract) *Anat. Rec.* 1: 58–59.

1907*b*. Observations on the living developing nerve fiber. *Anat. Rec.* 1: 116–18.

1908*a*. Regeneration of peripheral nerves. *Anat. Rec.* 1: 209.

1908*b*. Embryonic transplantation and development of the nervous system. *Anat. Rec.* 2: 385–410. (Harvey Lecture)

1910*a*. The development of peripheral nerve fibers in altered surroundings. *Arch. Entwicklungsmech. Organ.* 30: 15–33.

1910*b*. The outgrowth of the nerve fiber as a mode of protoplasmic movement. *J. Exp. Zool.* 9: 787–846.

1911. The stereotropism of embryonic cells. *Science* 34: 279–81.

1912. The cultivation of tissues in extraneous media as a method of morphogenetic study. *Anat. Rec.* 6: 181–93.

1913. Anatomy: Its scope, methods and relations to other biological sciences. *Anat. Rec.* 7: 401–10.

1914*a*. Science and practice. *Science* 40: 571–81.

1914*b*. The reaction of embryonic cells to solid structures. *J. Exp. Zool.* 17: 521–44.

1915. Experiments on the development of the limbs in Amphibia. *Proc. Nat. Acad. Sci.* 1: 539–44.

1916. On the reversal of laterality in the limbs of *Amblystoma* embryos. *Anat. Rec.* 10: 197–98.

1917. Transplantation of limbs. *Proc. Nat. Acad. Sci.* 3: 245–51.

1918. Experiments on the development of the fore limb of *Amblystoma*, a self-differentiating equipotential system. *J. Exp. Zool.* 25: 413–61.

1920. Experiments on the lens in *Amblystoma. Proc. Soc. Exp. Biol. Med.* 17: 199–200.

1921*a*. On relations of symmetry in transplanted limbs. *J. Exp. Zool.* 32: 1–136.

1921*b*. Experiments on the development of the gills in the amphibian embryo. *Biol. Bull.* 41: 156–70.

1924. Some unexpected results of the heteroplastic transplanation of limbs. *Proc. Nat. Acad. Sci.* 10: 69–74.

1925*a*. The development of the balancer in *Amblystoma*, studied by the method of transplantation and in relation to the connective-tissue problem. *J. Exp. Zool.* 41: 349–427.

1925*b*. The effect of reversing the medio-lateral or transverse axis of the forelimb bud in the salamander embryo (*Amblystoma punctatum Linn.*). *Arch. Entwicklungsmech. Organ.* 106: 469–502.

1925*c*. Heteroplastic transplantations of the eye in *Amblystoma*. *Anat. Rec.* 31: 299.

1929. Correlation in the development and growth of the eye studied by means of heteroplastic transplantation. *Arch. Entwicklungsmech. Organ.* 120: 1–55.

1931. Experiments on the development and growth of limbs in the Amphibia. *Science* 74: 575–76.

1933. Some difficulties of the determination problem. *Am. Nat.* 67: 306–21.

1935. Heteroplastic grafting in embryology. *Harvey Lectures*, 1933–34. Baltimore: Williams and Wilkins.

1936*a*. Relations of symmetry in the developing ear of *Amblystoma punctatum*. *Proc. Nat. Acad. Sci.* 22: 238–47.

1936*b*. Response on behalf of the medallist. *Science* 84: 565–67.

1937. Embryology and its relations. *Science* 85: 369–74.

1945. Facsimile of first announcement of the *Journal of Experimental Zoology*. Retrospect 1903–1945. *J. Exp. Zool.* 100: xi–xxxi.

1947. Wound healing and reconstitution of the central nervous system of the amphibian embryo after removal of parts of the neural plate. *J. Exp. Zool.* 106: 27–84.

1969. *Organization and Development of the Embryo*, ed. Sally Wilens. New Haven: Yale University Press.

Harrison, Ross G.; Astbury, W. T.; and Rudall, K. M.

1940. An attempt at an X-ray analysis of embryonic processes. *J. Exp. Zool.* 85: 339–63.

Hein, Hilde

1971. *On the Nature and Origin Of Life*. New York: McGraw-Hill.

1972. The endurance of the mechanism-vitalism controversy. *J. Hist. Biol.* 5: 159–88.

Henderson, L. J.

1913. *Fitness of the Environment*. New York: Macmillan.

1917. *Order of Nature*. Cambridge: Harvard University Press.

Hess, Eugene
  1969.   Origins of molecular biology. *Science* 168: 664–69.
Hesse, Mary
  1961.   *Forces and Fields*. London: Cambridge University Press.
  1966.   *Models and Analogies in Science*. South Bend, Ind.: University of Notre
          Dame Press.
Holtfreter, Johannes
  1939.   Gewebeaffinität, ein Mittel der embryonalen Formbildung. *Arch.
          Exp. Zellforsch.* 23: 169–209.
Huxley, J. S., and DeBeer, G. R.
  1934.   *The Elements of Experimental Embryology*. London: Cambridge
          University Press.
Jaeger, F. M.
  1917.   *Lectures on the Principles of Symmetry*. Amsterdam: Elsevier.
Japp, F. R.
  1898.   Stereochemistry and vitalism. *Chem. News* 27: 139–49.
Joravsky, David
  1972.   The head on Jung's pillow. *N. Y. Rev. Books* 19 (Sept. 21).
Karfunkel, Perry
  1971.   Experimental studies on the role of microtubules and microfilaments
          in neurulation. Ph.D. dissertation submitted to Yale University
          department of biology.
Kendrew, John C.
  1968.   Information and conformation in biology. In *Structural Chemistry and
          Molecular Biology: A Volume Dedicated to Linus Pauling by his Students,
          Colleagues, and Friends*. Alexander Rich and Norman Davidson (eds.).
          San Francisco: W. H. Freeman.
Koestler, Arthur
  1964.   *Act of Creation*. London: Hutchinson.
  1967.   *The Ghost in the Machine*. New York: Macmillan.
Koestler, A., and Smythies, J. R., eds.
  1969.   *Beyond Reductionism*. New York: Macmillan.
Köhler, Wolfgang
  1947.   *Gestalt Psychology*. New York: Liveright Publications.
Koltzov, N.
  1935.   *Physiologie du dévelopement et génétique*. Paris: Herman.
Kordig, Carl
  1971.   The theory-laddenness of observation. *Review of Metaphysics* 24:
          448–84.
Kuhn, Thomas
  1962.   *The Structure of Scientific Revolutions*. Chicago: Chicago University
          Press.

1970.   *The Structure of Scientific Revolutions*. 2nd ed. with postscript. Inter-
        national Encyclopedia of Science. Chicago: Chicago University
        Press.
Lakatos, I., and Musgrave, A., eds.
1970.   *Criticism and the Growth of Knowledge*. London: Cambridge University
        Press.
Lawrence, A. S. C.; Needham, J.; and Shih-Chang Shen
1944.   Studies on the anomalous viscosity and flow birefringence of protein
        solutions. I and II. *J. Gen. Physiol.* 27: 201–73.
Lenin, Vladimir Ilich
1927.   *Materialism and Empirico-criticism*. New York: International
        Publishers.
Liebig, Justus
1964.   *Animal Chemistry*, intro. Frederic L. Holmes. *The Sources of Science*, no.
        4. New York: Johnson Reprint.
Lillie, Ralph S., and Johnston, Earl N.
1919.   Precipitation-structures simulating organic growth. II. *Biol. Bull.*
        36: 225–72.
Loeb, Jacques
1964.   *The Mechanistic Conception of Life*, ed. Donald Fleming. Cambridge
        Mass.: Harvard University Press, Belknap Press.
Mach, Ernst
1942.   *The Science of Mechanics*, trans. Thomas J. McCormack, 5th ed.
        LaSalle, Illinois: Open Court Publishing.
McKie, D.
1944.   Wöhler's synthetic urea and the rejection of vitalism. *Nature* 153:
        609.
McPhearson, William
1917.   Asymmetric syntheses and their bearing upon the doctrine of
        vitalism. *Science* 45: 49–57, 76–81.
Mastermann, Margaret
1970.   The nature of a paradigm. In *Criticism and the Growth of Knowledge*.
        London: Cambridge University Press.
Mueller, Johannes
1839.   *Elements of Physiology*, trans. William Baly, 2nd ed. London: Taylor
        and Walton.
Nagel, Ernest
1951.   Mechanistic explanation and organismic biology. *Philosophy Phenom.*
        Res. 11: 327–38.
Needham, Dorothy M.
1972.   *Machina Carnis: The Biochemistry of Muscular Contraction in Its
        Historical Development*. London: Cambridge University Press.

Needham, Joseph

1923. Studies on inisotol. *Biochem. J.* 17: 422–30.

1924. Metabolic behavior of inisotol in the developing avian egg. *Biochem. J.* 18: 1371–80.

1925. The philosophical basis of biochemistry. *Monist* 35: 27–48.

1926a. The energy sources in ontogenesis. *Brit. J. Exp. Biol.* 3: 189–205.

1926b. The hydrogen-ion concentration and oxidation-reduction potential of the cell interior before and after fertilization and cleavage. *Proc. Roy. Soc. London, Ser. B* 99: 173–99.

1927. The free carbohydrate of the developing chick. *Quart. J. Exp. Physiol.* 18: 161–72.

1928a. *Man a Machine.* London: Kegan Paul.

1928b. Recent developments in the philosophy of biology. *Quart. Rev. Biol.* 3: 77–91.

1930a. The biochemical aspect of the recapitulation theory. *Biol. Rev.* 5: 142–58.

1930b. *The Sceptical Biologist.* New York: W. W. Norton.

1931. *Chemical Embryology*, 3 vols. London: Cambridge University Press. Reprint New York: Hafner, 1963.

1932. *The Great Amphibian.* London: Student Christian Movement Press.

1933a. A manometric analysis of the metabolism in avian ontogenesis. *Proc. Roy. Soc. London, Ser. B* 113: 429–59.

1933b. On the dissociability of the fundamental processes in ontogenesis. *Biol. Rev.* 8: 180–223.

1933c. The energy sources in ontogenesis. VII. The respiratory quotient of developing crustacean embryos. *J. Exp. Biol.* 10: 79–87.

1934a. *A History of Embryology.* London: Cambridge University Press.

1934b. Chemical heterogony and the ground plan of animal growth. *Biol. Rev.* 9: 79–109.

1936. *Order and Life.* New Haven: Yale University Press.

1937. Chemical aspects of morphogenetic fields. In *Perspectives in Biochemistry*, ed. J. Needham and D. E. Green. London: Cambridge University Press.

1941. Matter, form, evolution, and us. *This Changing World* 6: 15–22.

1942. *Biochemistry and Morphogenesis.* London: Cambridge University Press.

1943. *Time: The Refreshing River. Essays and Address*, 1932–42. New York: Macmillan.

1945. *History Is on Our Side.* London: Allen and Unwin.

1951. Biochemical aspects of form and growth. In *Aspects of Form*, ed. L. L. Whyte. Bloomington: Indiana University Press.

1962. Frederick Gowland Hopkins. *Perspect. Biol. Med.* 6: 2–47.

1968. Organizer phenomena after four decades: A retrospect. In *Haldane*

  and Modern Biology, ed. K. R. Dronamraju. Baltimore: Johns
  Hopkins University Press.
  Science and Civilization in China. 1954–71. 4 vols. in 5. London:
  Cambridge University Press.

Needham, J.; Waddington, C. H.; and Needham, Dorothy
 1934. Physico-chemical experiments on the amphibian organizer. *Proc.
  Roy. Soc. London, Ser. B* 114: 393–423.

Nicholas, J. S.
 1961. Ross Granville Harrison. *Nat. Acad. Sci., Biograph. Mem.* 35:
  130–62.

Olby, Robert
 1974. *The Path to the Double Helix.* London: Macmillan.

Oppenheimer, Jane M.
 1966. The growth and development of developmental biology. In *Major
  Problems in Developmental Biology*, ed. Michael Locke. New York:
  Academic Press.
 1967. *Essays in the History of Embryology and Biology.* Cambridge, Mass.:
  MIT Press.

Pantin, C. F. A.
 1968. *The Relations between the Sciences.* London: Cambridge University
  Press.

Pauling, Linus
 1970. Fifty years of progress in structural chemistry and molecular
  biology. In *The Making of Modern Science: Biographical Studies.
  Daedalus* 99: 988–1014.

Pauling, Linus, and Delbrück, Max
 1940. The nature of intermolecular forces operative in biochemical
  processes. *Science* 92: 77–99.

Pepper, Stephen
 1961. *World Hypotheses: A Study in Evidence.* Berkeley: University of
  California Press.

Piaget, Jean
 1967*a*. *Biologie et connaissance.* Paris: Gallimard.

Piaget, Jean, ed.
 1967*b*. *Logique et connaissance scientific.* Paris: Gallimard.

Piaget, Jean
 1971. *Structuralism*, trans. C. Maschler. New York: Harper and Row.

Polanyi, Michael
 1958. *Personal Knowledge.* Chicago: Chicago University Press.
 1966. *The Tacit Dimension.* New York: Doubleday.
 1968. Life's irreducible structure. *Science* 160: 1308–12.

Price, D. J. de Solla
 1973. Joseph Needham and the science of China. In *Chinese Science:*

Explorations of an Ancient Tradition, ed. S. Nakayama and N. Sivin, Cambridge, Mass.: MIT Press.

Prizbram, H.

   1906.   Kristall-Analogien zur Entwicklungsmechanik der Organismen. *Arch. Entwicklungsmech. Organ.* 22: 207–87.

Ritter, W. E.

   1919.   *The Unity of the Organism*, 2 vols. Boston: Gorham Press.

Ritterbush, Phillip

   1968.   *The Art of Organic Forms*. Washington: Smithsonian Institute Press.

Roux, Wilhelm

   1881.   *Der Kampf der Tiele im Organismus*. Leipzig: Wilhelm Engelmann.

   1885.   Beitrage zur Entwicklungsmechanik des Embryo. In *Gesammelt Abhandlungen über Entwicklungsmechanik der Organismen*. Vol. 1, pp. 257–76.

   1890.   *Die Entwicklungsmechanik der Organismen, eine anatomische Wissenschaft der Zukunft*. Vienna: Urban und Schwarzenberg.

   1923.   Wilhelm Roux in Halle an der Saale. In *Die Medizin der Gegenwart in Selbstdarstellungen*, ed. R. L. Grote. Vol. 1, pp. 141–206. Leipzig: Felix Meiner.

Rubner, Max

   1894.   Die Quelle der tierschen Wärme. *Z. Biol.* 30: 87–88.

Russell, E. S.

   1930.   *The Interpretation of Development and Heredity*. Oxford: Clarendon Press.

   1945.   *The Directiveness of Organic Activities*. London: Cambridge University Press.

Salm, Peter

   1971.   *The Poem as Plant: A Biological View of Goethe's Faust*. Cleveland: Case Western Reserve University Press.

Samuel, Edmund

   1972.   *Order: In Life*. Englewood Cliffs, N. J.: Prentice Hall.

Schaffner, Kenneth F.

   1967.   Antireductionism and molecular biology. *Science* 157: 644–47.

Schmidt, W. J.

   1924.   *Die Bausteine des Tierkörpers in polarisiertem Lichte*. Bonn: F. Cohen.

Schwann, Theodor

   1847.   *Microscopial Researches into the Accordance in the Structure and Growth of Animals and Plants*, trans. Henry Smith. London: Sydenham Society.

Science at the Crossroads

   1931.   Papers presented at the International Congress of the History of Science and Technology in London by delegates from the USSR. London: Kniga Press.

Simon, Michael A.
  1971.   *The Matter of Life*. New Haven: Yale University Press.
Spemann, Hans
  1938.   *Embryonic Development and Induction*. New Haven: Yale University
          Press.
Taylor, A. C.
  1943.   Development of the innervation pattern in the limb bud of the frog.
          Anat. Rec. 87: 379–413.
Thom, René
  1970.   Topological models in biology. In *Towards a Theoretical Biology,
          Drafts*, ed. C. H. Waddington. Edinburgh University Press.
Thompson, D'Arcy Wentworth
  1917.   *On Growth and Form*. London: Cambridge University Press.
Toulmin, Stephen
  1970.   Does the distinction between normal and revolutionary science
          hold water? In *Criticism and the Growth of Knowledge*. London:
          Cambridge University Press.
Toulmin, S., and Goodfield, J.
  1962.   *The Architecture of Matter*. London: Hutchinson.
Twitty, V. C.
  1966.   *Of Salamanders and Scientists*. San Francisco: W. H. Freeman.
Waddington, C. H.
  1934.   Morphogenetic fields. *Science Congress* 114: 336–46.
  1956.   *Principles of Embryology*. New York: Macmillan.
  1966.   Fields and gradients. In *Major Problems in Developmental Biology*, ed.
          Michael Locke. New York: Academic Press.
Waddington, C. H.; Needham, J.; and Brachet, Jean
  1936.   Studies on the nature of the amphibian organization center. III.
          The activation of the evocator. *Proc. Roy. Soc. London, Ser. B* 120:
          172–98.
Waddington, C. H.; Needham, J.; Nowinski, W. W.; Lemberg, Rudolf; and
Cohen, Arthur
  1936.   IV. Further experiments on the chemistry of the evocator. *Proc.
          Roy. London, Ser. B* 120: 198–208.
Watson, J. D.
  1965.   *Molecular Biology of the Gene*. New York: W. H. Benjamin.
Weiss, Paul
  1925a. Unabhängigkeit der Extremitätenregeneration vom Skelett (bei
          Triton cristatus). *Arch. Entwicklungsmech. Organ.* 104: 359–94.
  1925b. Tierisches Verhalten als "Systemreaktion." Die Orientierung der
          Ruhestellungen von Schmetterlingen (*Vanessa*) gegen Licht und
          Schwerkraft. *Biologia Gen.* 1: 168–248.

1926.   Morphodynamik. Ein Einblick in die Gesetze der organischen Gestaltung an Hand von experimentellen Ergebnissen. *Abhandlungen zur Theoretischen Biologie.* Vol. 23. Berlin: Verlag von Gebrüder Borntraeger.

1929.   Erzwingung elementarer Strukturverschiedenheiten am *in vitro* wachsenden Gewebe. Die Wirkung mechanischer Spannung auf Richtung und Intensität des Gewebewachstums und ihre Analyse. *Arch. Entwicklungsmech. Organ.* 116: 438–554.

1930.   *Entwicklungsphysiologie der Tiere.* Dresden und Leipzig: Steinkopff.

1934*a*.   Secretory activity of the inner layer of the embryonic mid-brain in the chick, as revealed by tissue culture. *Anat. Rec.* 58: 299–302.

1934*b*.   *In vitro* experiments on the factors determining the course of the outgrowing nerve fiber. *J. Exp. Zool.* 68: 393–448.

1935.   The so-called organizer and the problem of organization in amphibian development. *Physiol. Rev.* 15: 639–74.

1936.   Selectivity controlling the central-peripheral relations in the nervous system. *Biol. Rev.* 11: 494–531.

1939.   *Principles of Development.* New York: Holt, Rinehart, and Winston. Reprint New York: Hafner, 1969.

1940.   The problem of cell individuality in development. *Am. Nat.* 74: 34–46.

1941.   Nerve patterns: The mechanics of nerve growth. *Growth* 5: 163–203.

1942.   Lid-closure reflex from eyes transplanted to atypical locations in *Triturus torosus*: Evidence of a peripheral origin of sensory specificity. *J. Comp. Neurol.* 77: 131–69.

1944.   *In vitro* transformation of spindle cells of neural origin into macrophages. *Anat. Rec.* 88: 205–21.

1945.   Experiments on cell and axon orientation *in vitro*: The role of colloidal exudates in tissue organization. *J. Exp. Zool.* 100: 353–86.

1949.   Growth and differentiation on the cellular and molecular levels. *Proceedings of the 6th International Congress of Experimental Cytology*, pp. 475–82. New York: Academic Press.

1950*a*.   Experimental analysis of coordination by the disarrangement of central-peripheral relations. *Symp. Soc. Exp. Biol.* 4: 92–111.

1950*b*.   The outlook in morphogenesis. *Ann. Biol.* 26: 563–82.

1950*c*.   The deplantation of fragments of nervous system in amphibians. I. Central reorganization and the formation of nerves. *J. Exp. Zool.* 113: 397–461.

1955.   Beauty and the beast: Life and the rule of order. *Sci. Monthly* 81: 286–99.

1956.   The compounding of complex macromolecular and cellular units into tissue fabrics. *Proc. Nat. Acad. Sci.* 42: 819–30.

1957.   Macromolecular fabrics and patterns. *J. Cell. Comp. Physiol.* 49, Suppl. 1: 105–12.

1959.   Animal behavior as system reaction: Orientation toward light and gravity in the resting postures of butterflies (*Vanessa*). General Systems: *Yearbook for the Society for General Systems Research* 4: 1–44.

1960.   Ross Granville Harrison, 1870–1959, Memorial minute, *Rockefeller Institute Quarterly*, p. 6.

1964.   The dynamics of the membrane-bound incompressible body: A mechanism of cellular and subcellular motility. *Proc. Nat. Acad. Sci.* 52: 1024–29.

1965.   From cell dynamics to tissue architecture. In *Structure and Function of Connective and Skeletal Tissue*, pp. 256–63. London: Butterworths.

1967.   1 + 1 ≠ 2. (When one plus one does not equal two). In *The Neurosciences: A Study Program*, pp. 801–21. New York: Rockefeller University Press.

1968.   *Dynamics of Development: Experiments and Inferences.* New York: Academic Press.

1969.   The living system: Determinism stratified. *Studium Generale* 22: 361–400.

Weiss, Paul, and Amprino, Rudolfo

1940.   The effect of mechanical stress on the differentiation of scleral cartilage *in vitro* and in the embryo. *Growth* 4: 245–58.

Weiss, Paul, and Andres, Gert

1952.   Experiments on the fate of embryonic cells (chick) disseminated by the vascular route. *J. Exp. Zool.* 121: 449–87.

Weiss, Paul, and Ferris, Wayne

1954.   Electronmicroscopic study of the texture of the basement membrane of larval amphibian skin. *Proc. Nat. Acad. Sci.* 40: 528–40.

1956.   The basement lamella of amphibian skin: Its reconstruction after wounding. *J. Biophys. Biochem. Cytol.* 2: 275–82.

Weiss, Paul, and Garber, Beatrice

1952.   Shape and movement of mesenchyme cells as functions of the physical structure of the medium. Contributions to a quantitative morphology. *Proc. Nat. Acad. Sci.* 38: 264–80.

Weiss, Paul, and Grover, Norman

1968.   Helical arrays of polyribosomes. *Proc. Nat. Acad. Sci.* 59: 763–68.

Weiss, Paul, and Hiscoe, H. B.

1948.   Experiments on the mechanism of nerve growth. *J. Exp. Zool.* 107: 315–95.

Weiss, Paul, and James, Ruth

1955*a*. Aberrant (circular) myofibrils in amphibian larvae: An example of orthogonal tissue structure. *J. Exp. Zool.* 129: 607–22.

1955*b*. Skin metaplasia *in vitro* induced by brief exposure to Vitamin A. *Exp. Cell Res.*, Suppl. 3: 381–94.

Weiss, Paul, and Kavanau, Lee

    1957. A model of growth and growth control in mathematical terms. *J. Gen. Physiol.* 41: 1–47.

Weiss, Paul, and Moscona, Aron

    1958. Type-specific morphogenesis of cartilages developed from dissociated limb and scleral mesenchyme *in vitro*. *J. Embryol. Exp. Morph.* 6: 238–46.

Weiss, Paul, and Scott, Bruce I. H.

    1963. Polarization of cell locomotion *in vitro*. *Proc. Nat. Acad. Sci.* 50: 330–36.

Weiss, Paul, and Taylor, A. C.

    1944. Further experimental evidence against "neurotropism" in nerve regeneration. *J. Exp. Zool.* 95: 233–57.

    1960. Reconstitution of complete organs from single-cell suspensions of chick embryos in advanced stages of differentiation. *Proc. Nat. Acad. Sci.* 46: 1177–85.

Werskey, P. G.

    1970. Socialist scientists in Britain, 1918–40; The Visible College. Dissertation in progress, Harvard University, Cambridge, Massachusetts.

Whitehead, A. N.

    1925. *Science and the Modern World.* New York: Macmillan.

    1929. *Process and Reality.* New York: Macmillan.

Willier, B.; Weiss, P.; and Hamburger, V., eds.

    1955. *Analysis of Development.* Philadelphia: W. B. Saunders.

Wilson, E. B.

    1896. *The Cell in Development and Inheritance. The Sources of Science*, no. 30. New York: Johnson Reprint, 1966.

Wolpert, Lewis

    1970. Positional information and pattern formation. In *Towards a Theoretical Biology, Drafts*, ed. C. H. Waddington. Edinburgh: Edinburgh University Press.

Woodger, J. H.

    1929. *Biological Principles.* New York: Harcourt, Brace.

    1930*a* and 1931. The "concept of organism" and the relation between embryology and genetics. *Quart. Rev. Biol.* 5: 1–22, 438–63; 6: 178–95.

    1930*b*. Review of *The Sceptical Biologist. Mind* 39: 244–246.

Wrinch, Dorothy

    1938. Is there a protein fabric? *Cold Spring Harbor Symp. Quant. Biol.* 6: 122–39.

Index

Aesthetic sense, 16, 42, 111*n*
Alexander, Samuel, 37
Alpbach Symposium, 5, 183–84. *See also* Paradigm community
Amblystoma: studies on balancer system, 79–81; studies on limb system, 65, 73–77
Analogy: logical status of, 9; between plant form and fabric, 41; from physics applied to biology, 59; importance of in biology, 84, 189. *See also* Metaphor
Analysis: Harrison's approach, 64; importance of, 84; limits of, 185
Anatomy: Harrison's ideas on, 42–44; relation to physiology, 44
Arber, Agnes, 42
Architecture: in connective tissue, 168
Aristotle: Driesch's debt to, 23; in lineage of organicists, 37; use of art-artisan-organism analogy, 40; use of architectural principles, 41; Harrison's relation to, 44; Needham's discussion of, 128–129; treatment of form, 171*n;* justification for study of living things, 188
Arrhenius, Svante, 21
Art: relation to biology, 40, 41, 47–48
Artefact paradigm, 189
Astbury, William Thomas: study of textile fibers, 46; crystallographic studies with Harrison, 81–82; influence on Harrison, 91; X-ray analysis of protein structure, 91
Asymmetry: as basis of vitalism, 48; protein structure in explanation of, 90–91. *See also* Symmetry; Vitalism
Atomism, 20
Autonomy: of biology, 26*n,* 174–75, 195; of a science, 194
Axiomatization: importance to reduction, 195

Bacon, Francis, 18

Bacteriology, 65, 71
Baer, Karl Ernst von: importance for analytical embryology, 28; as organicist, 34–35; biological philosophy of, 36
Baitsell, George, 89*n*
Beckner, Morton, 33
Beer, Gavin de, 53, 53*n*
Bernal, J. D.: as socialist scientist, 21*n;* source of Needham's crystal terminology, 133
Bernard, Claude, 35, 36
Bertalanffy, Ludwig von: organicism of, 26, 27, 38, 63*n;* debt to Weiss, 38*n;* systems thinking of, 38*n;* as structuralist-organicist, 63; introduction of *Gestalt-prinzip,* 114; participant in Alpbach Symposium, 184
Bichât, Marie François Xavier, 36
Biochemistry, 44*n,* 119*n*
Biogen, 108
Biological laws: autonomy of, 194, 197, 198
Biological level: investigation on, 79, 140. *See also* Hierarchy; Organization
Biology: relation to physics, 4, 83, 86, 112, 114, 186, 194; relation to art, 41, 47–48; Weiss's subcategorization of, 182*n*
Black, Max, 9–10, 133*n*
Boell, E. J., 122–23
Bohr, Niels: indeterminacy in biology, 140
Born, Gustav: method of embryonic transplantation of, 65–66, 99
Boundaries, 63, 80. *See also* Organization; Structure
Boveri, Theodor: importance of gradients for, 52–53; visual images for, 53*n*
Boyle, Robert, 18
Braus, Hermann, 69–70
Brooks, William Keith: students of, 13, 36, 65, 65*n*
Brücke, Ernst, 20

221